THE VEGAN ATHLETE

Plant-Based Nutrition and High-Protein Meals for Vegan Athletes and Bodybuilders

- Mark Power -

© Copyright 2020 by Mark Power - All rights reserved.

This Book is provided with the sole purpose of providing relevant information on a specific topic for which every reasonable effort has been made to ensure that it is both accurate and reasonable. Nevertheless, by purchasing this Book you consent to the fact that the author, as well as the publisher, are in no way experts on the topics contained herein, regardless of any claims as such that may be made within. As such, any suggestions or recommendations that are made within are done so purely for entertainment value. It is recommended that you always consult a professional prior to undertaking any of the advice or techniques discussed within.
This is a legally binding declaration that is considered both valid and fair by both the Committee of Publishers Association and the American Bar Association and should be considered as legally binding within the United States.
The reproduction, transmission, and duplication of any of the content found herein, including any specific or extended information will be done as an illegal act regardless of the end form the information ultimately takes. This includes copied versions of the work both physical, digital and audio unless express consent of the Publisher is provided beforehand. Any additional rights reserved.
Furthermore, the information that can be found within the pages described forthwith shall be considered both accurate and truthful when it comes to the recounting of facts. As such, any use, correct or incorrect, of the provided information will render the Publisher free of responsibility as to the actions taken outside of their direct purview. Regardless, there are zero scenarios where the original author or the Publisher can be deemed liable in any fashion for any damages or hardships that may result from any of the information discussed herein.
Additionally, the information in the following pages is intended only for informational purposes and should thus be thought of as universal. As befitting its nature, it is presented without assurance regarding its prolonged validity or interim quality. Trademarks that are mentioned are done without written consent and can in no way be considered an endorsement from the trademark holder.

Table of Contents

INTRODUCTION 7

PART 1 - VEGAN DIET FOR ATHLETES 11

CHAPTER 1: WHAT IS THE VEGAN DIET? 13
    TYPES OF VEGAN DIETS 14
    THE HEALTH BENEFITS 16
    EATING ON THE VEGAN DIET 17
    ARE THERE RISKS? 18

CHAPTER 2: WHY DOES PROTEIN MATTER? 21

CHAPTER 3: HOW TO GET THE RIGHT NUTRITION FOR ANAEROBIC ACTIVITY 25

CHAPTER 4: WHY BODYBUILDERS SHOULD CONSIDER THE VEGAN DIET 29

PART II - RECIPES AND MEAL PLANS TO FUEL YOUR WORKOUTS 35

CHAPTER 5: THE MEAL PLAN 37

CHAPTER 6: WORKOUT BREAKFASTS 39
    Blueberry Muffins 39
    Banana Bread 40
    Pancakes 41
    Pecan and Maple Granola 42
    Overnight Oatmeal 43
    Pumpkin Pie Oatmeal 44
    Peanut Butter and Chocolate Quinoa 45
    Early Morning Scramble 46
    Loaded Breakfast Burrito 47
    Sweet Potato Skillet 49
    Vegan Omelet 50

CHAPTER 7: SAUCES AND DIPS 53
BBQ Sauce 53
Your Own Marinara Sauce 54
Taco Salsa 55
Apple Sauce 56
Vegan Mayo 57
Easy Enchilada Sauce 58

CHAPTER 8: EASY LUNCH RECIPES 59
BBQ Sliders 59
Hawaiian Burgers 60
Falafel Burgers 62
Vegan Pizza Bread 64
Baked Mac and Peas 65
Sweet Potato Casserole 66
Sunday Roast 67
Vegetable Stir-Fry 68
Vegetable Spring Rolls with Sauce 69
Orange Tofu Bowl 71
Mango Chickpea Curry 73
Italian Bean Balls 74
Crispy Chicken Salad 76
Arugula and Lentil Salad 77
Quinoa and Vegetables 79
Chickpea Sunflower Sandwich 80
Chickpea and Lentil Bowl 82
Vegan Chicken, Tomato and Lettuce Sandwich 83
Tempeh and Carrot Salad 84
Kidney Bean and Feta Cheese Salad 86
Lentil Salad 88

CHAPTER 9: DINNER RECIPES 90
Vegan Enchiladas 90
Tex-Mex Tofu with Beans 92
Tofu Cacciatore 94
Mushroom Stroganoff 96
BBQ Grits and Greens 98
Easy Burritos 100

Fajitas *102*
Farro Protein Bowls *104*
Seitan Wings *106*
Easy Dinner Tacos *108*
Grilled Tofu Steaks *110*
Vegan Hot Dogs *111*
Sausage and Tomato Pasta *112*
Mongolian Seitan *114*
Vegan Burgers *116*
Lentil Loaf with BBQ *117*
Lentil Ragu *119*
Seitan and Black Bean Stir Fry *121*
Vegan Sausage Rolls *123*
Spicy Rice in One Pan *125*
Vegan Banh Mi *126*
Curried Tofu Wraps *127*

CHAPTER 10: SNACKS AND DESSERTS **128**
Chocolate Chip Muffins *128*
Black Bean and Chocolate Pudding *129*
Hazelnut and Chocolate Bars *130*
Sweet Lentil Bites *131*
No-Bake Treats *133*
Zucchini Muffins *134*
Lemon Bars *136*
Sunflower Protein Bars *137*
Southwest Stuffed Bowls *138*
Brownie Bars *139*
Chewy Butter Balls *140*
Carrot Cake *141*
Protein Oat and Banana Balls *143*
Protein Brownies *144*
Oatmeal Raisin Cookies *145*

CONCLUSION **147**

Introduction

Congratulations on purchasing *The Vegan Athlete,* and thank you for doing so.

The following chapters will discuss all of the different parts of the vegan diet that you need to know in order to be successful as an athlete. When we think about the traditional athlete, especially when we are talking about those who spend time weight lifting and doing other strenuous kinds of exercises, we think of a completely different diet plan. We assume that the vegan diet is going to lack a lot of the important nutrients and the other things that these athletes need. But as we will find in this guidebook, the vegan diet may be the perfect choice for these athletes if they want to fill up with the best foods, while ensuring that they can get their best performance ever as well.

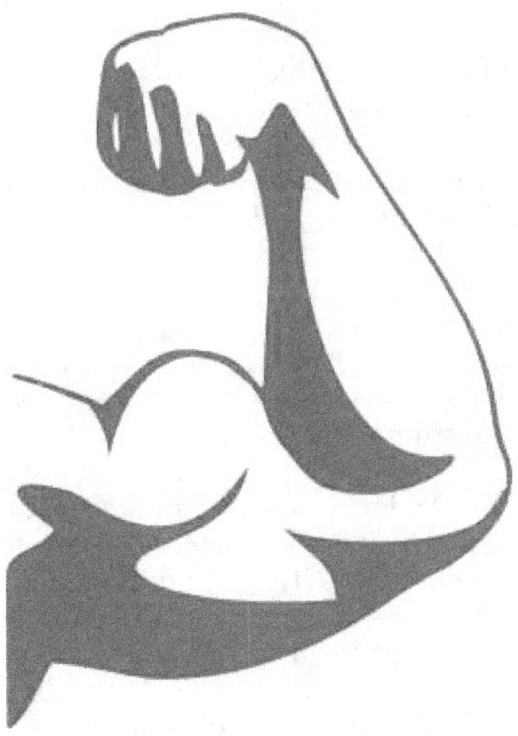

There are a lot of topics about the vegan diet for athletes, and we are going to take some time to explore as many of them as possible in this guidebook. We are going to start out with a little look at the vegan diet and what it is all about. We can talk about the basics, some of the rules for eating on this diet, and even a look at some of the health benefits and more of following this diet plan. The vegan diet, when it is done with whole and plant-based food and not with a bunch of junk that is labeled as vegan, can be one of the healthiest diet plans around, and we are going to take a look at how this is so.

When that is done, it is time for us to move on to some of the other things that we need to know when it comes to the vegan diet and using it for the athletes we know. We are going to take a look at how the protein that is found in our diets is so important and how the vegan diet is able to meet this, even for the bodybuilder and the athlete. Then we will have a discussion about anaerobic exercise and some of the unique nutritional requirements of these individuals, with a discussion of how the vegan diet will be able to meet those as well.

While the topics above are going to be very important, we are also going to take some time to explore how the vegan diet is going to be able to help us out as bodybuilders. We will look at how bodybuilders, in particular, are able to benefit from this kind of diet plan and some of the simple adjustments that we need to make to this diet plan to ensure that the bodybuilder is able to increase their performance, see the best results, and still get the healthy nutrition that they need.

When we are done taking a look at all of the great things about the vegan diet and why it is so amazing, it is time to dive into some of the delicious recipes that we are able to utilize here. There is so much to love about the vegan diet, and it is so important for us to see how tasty and delicious it can be, even for someone who is a beginner in using it, and for someone who is an athlete. We will include a ton of recipes for breakfast, lunch, dinner, dessert, snacks and more, and some of the nutritional information so you can make the best decisions for your meal planning needs.

As we can see, there are a ton of things to discuss when it comes to the vegan diet for athletes, and this guidebook is going to attempt to go through many of them so you can see that this is the best choice for you. When you are ready to get started on the vegan diet and you want to see how this can work for your needs, make sure to check out this guidebook to help you get started.

There are plenty of books on this subject on the market, thanks again for choosing this one! Every effort was made to ensure it is full of as much useful information as possible. Please enjoy it!

PART 1
VEGAN DIET FOR ATHLETES

Chapter 1: What is the Vegan Diet?

No matter what your goals are, whether you are trying to crush your weight loss, you are trying to improve your heart health, cut down on blood pressure, or even fight off diabetes, you will need to choose a strong and effective diet plan to help you make this happen. And one of the healthiest, and the most popular, diet plans that are available for us to try now is known as the vegan diet.

When the vegan diet is done in the right manner, it is going to result in a lot of great health benefits. It can help the participant to get a lot more nutrients than they may be taking in with their traditional diet. It is going to help improve some of the control that the individual has on their blood sugar levels, and it can result in a trimmer waistline. You have to be careful to not go through and eat too many of the same foods, or you are going to run into trouble with nutrient deficiencies. But when you do it well, you will not run into issues at all.

Veganism is going to be a method of living that is going to try and exclude and take out all forms possible of animal exploitation and cruelty, whether for clothing, food, or any of the other purposes that are there. For these reasons and more, this kind of diet plan is going to be devoid of all animal products. This includes dairy, eggs, and meat.

There are a number of reasons why someone would choose to go on this kind of diet plan. The first reason is for their health. This is a great way to lose weight, improve your heart health, and so much more. Others are going to do it for environmental concerns and some do it for ethics. There are a lot of reasons why people will choose to go on a diet plan like the vegan diet, and you can choose the reason that works the best for us.

TYPES OF VEGAN DIETS

There are actually a few different versions of the vegan diet that someone is able to follow. Most of them can be healthy and good for your health, though a few are going to be a little bit questionable here, and you have to consider whether they are actually any better than the regular diet that you were on before. Some of the choices that you can make when it comes to the vegan diet will include:

1. **The whole-food vegan diet**. This is going to take some time to look at a lot of whole foods and have the participant eat mostly those. This is going to include lots of seeds, nuts, legumes, whole grains, and of course, a lot of fresh produce in order to get the nutrients that you need.
2. **The junk food vegan diet**. This is a version that you can go on, and you are sure to find a bunch of junk food that is technically vegan. But you will not lose a bit of weight because it is going to be full of fake and processed foods rather than the foods that are actually good for you and can help you to lose weight. You should stay away from this option as much as possible if you want to keep your health in line.
3. **Raw food vegan diet**. This is going to be the version of the diet that will still stick with a lot of healthy and whole foods but will require that we do not cook any of these at temperatures that are higher than 118 degrees at all.
4. **The thrive diet**. This is going to be one of the versions of the raw food vegan diet. Those who decide to follow

this are going to eat a lot of whole foods that are based on plants that are going to be minimally cooked at some really low temperatures or that will be raw in the process.
5. **80/10/10**. With this diet plan, you are going to eat raw food vegan and limit your plants that are higher in fats, including nuts and sometimes avocados. This one can often be known as the fruitarian diet and will rely on soft greens and raw fruits instead.
6. **Raw until 4**. This is going to be a diet that is similar to what we talked about above, but it is going to change it up a bit and make it easier for some people to follow. With this one, you are going to consume a lot of raw foods until 4 in the afternoon. Then you have the option to cook up a meal that is based on plants for your dinner in the evening.
7. **The starch solution**. This one is going to focus a bit more on the cooked starches like rice and corn and potatoes and a bit less on the fruits that you want to eat.

Although there are going to be a lot of variations to the vegan diet that you are able to follow, you will find that they can all lead to a healthier method of eating than what you did in the past. This can be good news for those who are just getting started along the way. But keep in mind that most of the scientific research out there about this kind of diet plan will just focus n the vegan diet as a whole, and hasn't been able to look at each of these on their own.

We have to remember that if we want to get all of the great benefits that are out there for the vegan diet, then we need to eat foods that are wholesome and good for us. There are a lot of fake products that are technically vegan, but they have been so processed and changed that they are not going to be good for us. If we make our vegan diet have just those foods, then we are technically vegan, but we are not getting the wholesome and good foods with all of the nutrients, and then we will not get the health benefits that we are looking for.

There are a lot of things to love when it comes to working with the vegan diet, and it is likely that you are going to fall in love with it in no time as well! It has all of the healthy ingredients that you need and so much more that will help you to feel good, gain the muscles that you want, and so much more!

THE HEALTH BENEFITS

In addition to helping athletes to get healthier and see some of the best results possible with the workouts they are doing, there are a lot of other health benefits that we are able to see along the way as well. The vegan diet is often seen as one of the healthiest diet plans out there for people to try, and there are a lot of benefits of going with this one compared to some of the others.

Because you are getting rid of a lot of the foods that are considered unhealthy, and because you are cutting out the bad fats, the sodium, and the processed foods and sugars, you are automatically helping your body to get all of the good nutrients that it is looking for rather than all of the bad.

Most of us can agree that the traditional American diet is not going to be all that healthy to follow. It may seem like a good idea to start, but it is going to be a mess on our bodies. It causes us to gain weight, can make it hard to keep our hearts nice and strong, and can cause a whole host of other problems in the process as well. It may taste good and be really convenient to follow, but it is not healthy, and it is making it hard to do well as an athlete.

This is why the vegan diet can be so healthy. We are replacing all of that bad stuff that we just talked about with some of the good and healthy foods that our bodies need in the process. You get to eat a lot of good whole grains, fruits and vegetables, and healthy fats that are going to be so amazing overall for helping you to look and feel your best overall. And because of this, you get the benefit of having some really healthy and good health benefits as well.

Those who have gone on the vegan diet, and eaten the healthy version without all of the junk, have found that this is one of the best ways to lose weight, improve the health of the heart by lowering cholesterol and blood pressure, can help individuals to fight off issues with diabetes, and so much more in the process of following this kind of diet plan. It is as simple as that. You work to fill your body with lots of healthy foods and produce and things that are good for it, then it will learn how to heal and can do a much better job when it is time to perform in the manner that you would like.

EATING ON THE VEGAN DIET

Before you are able to start out with any kind of diet plan, it is important for us to go through and be prepared with the right kind of eating plan here. We need to make sure that we are consuming the right foods and avoiding the wrong foods in the process. The easiest way to remember what you are not allowed to consume on the vegan diet is that you can't have any animal products at all.

What this means is that you need to keep out all of the meat and the poultry that was found in your regular diet. This would be the goose, turkey chicken beef pork, lamb ad so on. We also need to keep out all of the seafood and the fish, so anything that comes out of the sea needs to be avoided here as well. The meat part of this is pretty easy to understand and follow so we don't need to spend a lot of time on this.

However, there are a few other groups of foods that need to be avoided when you are going with this kind of diet plan. Things like dairy, eggs, and beef products are all on the list of foods that need to be avoided. These come from animals, and so they are considered animal products. There are vegan kinds of milk and cheeses that you can use to replace these if needed and there are other vegan-friendly eggs that you can make, so don't feel like you need to avoid these completely. There are other animal-based ingredients that you have to be careful about as well including lactose, whey and more.

Now that we have listed out a lot of the things that you have to avoid when you are going through the vegan diet in order to get the best results from it. This is going to make you feel like there is nothing you are allowed to eat at all, and like you are lost for what will work or not. The good news is that once you get over the idea that there are a few things that you can't eat on this diet plan there are a lot of great-tasting and delicious foods that are completely allowed and you will still have a ton of tasty and delicious meals to enjoy on a regular basis.

There are many foods that we are able to enjoy, including some seitan, tempeh, and tofu that will provide us with a lot of protein. Legumes are good for a bit of protein and can provide us with a lot of other nutrients along with nuts, nut kinds of butter, and seeds. As we mentioned before, there are calcium-fortified yogurts and milk that are not dairy-based, such as cashew yogurt, so we can still get that vitamin B12 and D and the calcium for as long as we need.

Some of the other things that we are able to enjoy and eat plenty of when we are on the vegan diet will include things like nutritional yeast, whole grains, and other products that are made out of the whole grains, fermented and sprouted plant foods, and of course, lots of vegetables and fruits along the way as well.

ARE THERE RISKS?

There are a few risks with this diet plan when it comes to nutritional deficiencies along the way. Sometimes when we are changing over to this kind of diet plan and working on getting it all right and ensuring that we eat the right amounts and the right types of foods, deficiencies are going to show up on occasion. The good news though is if you do some meal planning and add a lot of variety to your meals, and you stick with the healthy foods and not all of the junk, even this is not going to be a problem. It may take a bit of trial and error to ensure that you can eat the right foods at the right times, but it evens out.

If you are worried about the nutritional deficiencies when you first get started, then the best option is to start taking a multivitamin. This is going to be perfect for ensuring that you are able to get a lot of the important nutrients in as you make the adjustments. As you get more used to the vegan diet, this will not be as big of a problem and you can stop taking the multivitamin if you would like and just focus on the healthy and wholesome foods instead.

There are a lot of great things to love when it comes to working with a vegan diet. It is a simple diet plan that allows us to eat foods that are wholesome and good for us, instead of eating all of the trash that is usually found on the traditional American diet. Following this kind of diet plan can help increase our performance, makes it easier to lose weight, and can be good for so many other aspects of our health. When you want a diet plan that is able to do it all, then the vegan diet is the right one to go with.

Chapter 2: Why Does Protein Matter?

When it comes to your athletic performance, there are a lot of different options and macronutrients that you need to consider. These are going to be so important to ensure that the body has all of the building blocks that it needs to stay healthy and happy for the long-term and not get sick in the process either. But one of the macronutrients that we need to focus on, and seems to be a topic of a lot of discussions when it comes to the vegan diet, is protein.

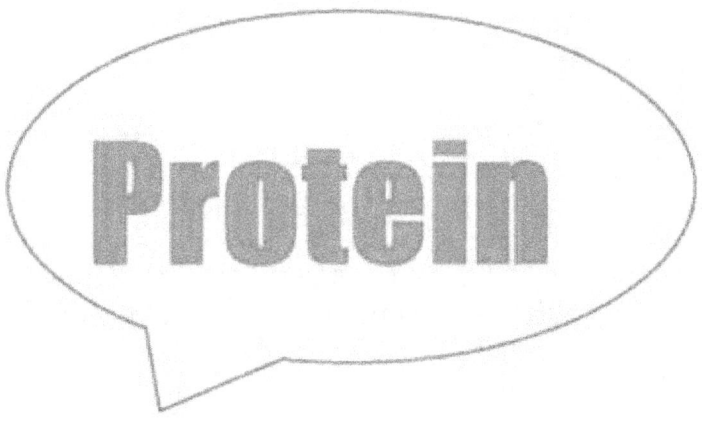

High-protein diets are going to be a really great thing when it comes to being a bodybuilder and trying to keep up with all of your athletic events. It is pretty common to see those who are on a diet grabbing some protein bars to help them to feel full and satisfied, and it is common for bodybuilders to take in several protein-shakes to help them go.

There is a lot of power behind this nutrient, and it is pretty easy to see where some of the excitement of consuming this and getting enough is going to come from. Protein is going to be such an important component that is seen in pretty much all of the cells of the body. Your nails and hair are going to be made up mostly of protein. Your body is able to utilize this protein to build up and repair the tissues when it is needed. It is also possible to use this protein to make hormones, enzymes, and some of the other chemicals that are important in the body. Protein is going to be one of the building blocks of the blood, skin, cartilage, muscles and bones.

Along with carbs and fat, protein is one of the macronutrients that the body needs. This means that our body actually needs a relatively large amount of it to function properly. Minerals and vitamins, which we need but in a much smaller amount, are going to be known as micronutrients. But unlike carbs and fat, the body is not going to hold onto and store protein, which means that we are not going to have a good reservoir around to draw on later if it is needed.

Many people assume that this means they need to eat protein all day long. But this is not the truth. We actually need less protein than we think, even though most of us can benefit from getting our protein from better food sources. We have all heard in the past that getting extra protein is able to build up more muscle. But the only way to build up the muscle that we want is through lots of exercises. Bodies need to have a modest amount of protein to go through and function well. The extra protein is not going to come in and give us extra strength.

There are a number of rules that we are able to follow in order to help us get the moderate amounts of protein that we need.

1. Teenage boys that are active are able to get the majority of protein that they need with three daily servings for a total of seven ounces.
2. Children between the ages of 2 to 6 and most women, along with some of the elderly, will get what they need when they have two daily servings for a total of five ounces.

3. And for active women, most men, teen girls, and older children, the guidelines are going to be closer to two daily servings to end up being six ounces.

So for most people, eating an eight-ounce steak is going to be enough to give you the protein that your body needs and more. You should find some better options here though. Steak is going to include a lot of the unhealthy saturated fats as well, and it is not allowed on the vegan diet to start with.

However, it is still important to make sure that we are taking in enough protein on a regular basis to help us to stay strong and to build up muscles. We don't need to just eat protein all day long, but adding some more into our diet plan will help us out so much. Some of the most important functions that we are able to see when we add more protein into our bodies include:

1. Maintenance and growth: Your body needs to have a lot of protein to help tissues to grow and stay strong. Under normal circumstances, the body is going to break down the same amount of protein that it will use to repair and build up tissue. But then there will be times when the body will break down more protein than it is able to create, such as while pregnant and when sick. Taking in more protein during this time can be important.
2. Can cause some biochemical reactions: Enzymes are going to be some proteins that will help to aid in all of the biochemical reactions that will take place in and out of your cells. These can help out with a lot of different things including the contractions of muscles, blood clotting, energy protection, and digestion.
3. It can be a messenger: It is possible for proteins to become hormones so that they are the chemical messengers that will aid in the communication between the organs, tissues, and cells. They are going to be made and then secreted through the glands and endocrine tissues and then your blood can move them around to reach their goal and send the message.

4. It can provide structure. Some of the proteins that you are able to work with are fibrous and can provide our tissues and cells with stiffness and the rigidity that it needs. Some of the proteins that we want to work with here include elastin, collagen, and keratin, which can help us to form some of the connective frameworks of certain structures in the body.
5. It can help to bolster the immune systems. Proteins are going to help us to form some immunoglobulins, which are known as antibodies, to fight infections. Antibodies are just going to be proteins that go to your blood to help make sure that your body is protected against viruses and bacteria. The more protein that you have in your body and the ore it is used well, the less likely you are to get sick.
6. It can help to transport and store all of the nutrients you need. This can include a lot of nutrients like oxygen, cholesterol, blood sugar, and various minerals and vitamins. Protein transporters are going to be really specific, which means that they are just going to bind to some specific substances and nothing else.
7. It can provide us with more energy: It is possible that protein is going to help us to get energy and to keep on moving during our workouts. But we do have to remember that the last thing our body will use up for energy is protein because it is a valuable nutrient and so many parts of the body use it. This is why we usually rely on fats and carbs to keep us going.

As we can already guess, there are a lot of benefits of working with protein and a bodybuilder or athlete will be able to enjoy a lot of them along the way. Being able to utilize the protein and get enough on the vegan diet is usually easier than it may seem, as long as we plan out our meals well and don't eat a lot of junk in the process. Even without the animal products, there are options that will allow us to go through and get the protein that we need, which can be great news overall.

Chapter 3: How to Get the Right Nutrition for Anaerobic Activity

When you are a bodybuilder, it is important to go through and make sure that you are eating a healthy diet the whole time. This will ensure that you are able to get all of the nutrition that you need, and can make it a whole lot easier for you to stay healthy and happy over the long-term as well. getting the right nutrition for this kind of activity is a bit of a challenge, and sometimes you will find that some of the other diet plans are not going to meet the nutrition values as you would like. But we are going to take some time in this chapter to look at the best ways that we can follow the vegan diet and provide our bodies with the right nutrition for anaerobic activity.

You will find that your body is able to reach an anaerobic state when you are able to work at the near-maximum effort. This means doing something like sprinting as fast you can for 400 meters or doing a short set of repetitions with a real heavyweight. You are not able to sustain this kind of state for a long time, so a workout that is anaerobic is going to include a series of lifts or sprints with minimal recovery that happens between them. When you do this, your body is able to convert the carbs that are present into quick energy, which is why they should be one of the main focuses when you plan the meal you want to eat before these workouts.

Carbs

This is why we need to focus on carbs. Unlike during some of the slower and the more moderate exercises that you want to do, where your body is able to convert some of the stored fat into fuel, these workouts are going to require a really fast source of fuel to get it done. The glycogen that is stored in your liver and your muscles, which is going to be there mainly from the carbs that you eat before the workout, is going to be easy to digest and can provide us with the fuel that we need.

Think back to the vegan diet and some of the amazing parts that are going to show up with it. There are a lot of benefits of choosing this kind of diet plan, and the best part is that there are a ton f healthy carbs that you are able to eat, including the whole grains and all of that healthy produce along the way. This means that you are more likely to get the carbs that you need to do these anaerobic exercises in no time when you are on the vegan diet.

During some of the shorter bursts of the high-intensity work, your body is able to convert some of the glycogen that is stored and some of the carbs that were recently consumed and then turn it into ATP and into creatine phosphate. This combination is going to provide us with the system for fuel for all activity.

With this in mind, we have to remember that it is important to stay away from some things like protein, fat, and fiber right before the workout. These are great additions to have in your diet during the rest of the day, but shortly before we go through one of the anaerobic exercises that we want to use, we need to make sure that we are avoiding these and keeping them out of our meals as much as possible.

Although whole grains are amazing and they are going to provide us with a lot of nutritional benefits, they are going to contain a lot of fiber, which is going to slow down how quickly the carbs are able to go through the digestion process. If you take on too much fiber in the few hours before this kind of workout, you may not end up with the access that you need to that fuel source, and it could end up with a lot of digestive distress in the process.

When you are creating your own pre-workout meal, you need to stick with some of the carbs that are a bit easier to digest and eat up. This would be the white bread and the sugars. Having too much protein and fat before the workout can cause a similar kind of effect on the body when it comes to your digestion and energy levels because your body needs to go through a complex process before it is able to turn these nutrients into fuel. A little protein and fat in the meal before a workout are fine, but you do need to keep it to a minimum rather than letting it be the main event all of the time.

While we are on the subject, we need to talk about the timing of your meal before the workout. If you have a meal that falls three to four hours before you plan to exercise, you are able to have a full meal that will have around 300 to 500 calories on it. Some of the things that you may want to try out here include something like a bagel, a nice salad with some tempeh or seitan on it, or a potato that has some cashew yogurt or salsa on it.

If you are only an hour or two from the workout, then we need to shrink the portion size a bit so that we are not still digesting it all. You could go with a cup of cashew yogurt, a fruit smoothie, or even a piece of fruit to get the energy that you need. And if your workout is even closer, say within half an hour, then going with a sports gel, a sports drink, or an apple can be what you need to get the carbs and the energy that you need to finish up this kind of workout.

Unlike some of the athletes out there who work more on endurance, the anaerobic athletes will not really need to focus on carb-loading at all. This idea of carb loading is going to involve eating a higher percentage, sometimes as high as 70 to 75 percent of our daily calories, from carbs for a few days before a competition or a big workout. The reason that some athletes will do this is to help them maximize the stores of energy that are found int heir muscles.

This is not something that really needs to be done in an anaerobic workout. These are going to utilize some of the glycogen that is stored in the muscles, but it is unlikely that you are going to go through and deplete the stores so much that you won't have any let because the workouts are going to be so small and will not last all that long.

Anaerobic exercise is going to work in a slightly different manner than what we are able to find, and we need to eat in a different manner than we would with some of the other forms of working out and exercising that you may have heard about in the past. Knowing the best ways to eat and being prepared for this will ensure that we are able to take care of our bodies and eat the right foods at the right times, and the vegan diet is able to step in and help make this work out great.

Chapter 4: Why Bodybuilders Should Consider the Vegan Diet

When we hear about the vegan diet and the word bodybuilding, we are going to be a bit confused. It is not often that the two of these are going to come together and be used in the same sentence, much less actually be things that we are able to do together. But there are a growing number of bodybuilders who are jumping in on the idea of going on the vegan diet and using this as a way to help them to tone up and get the healthy nutrients that they need.

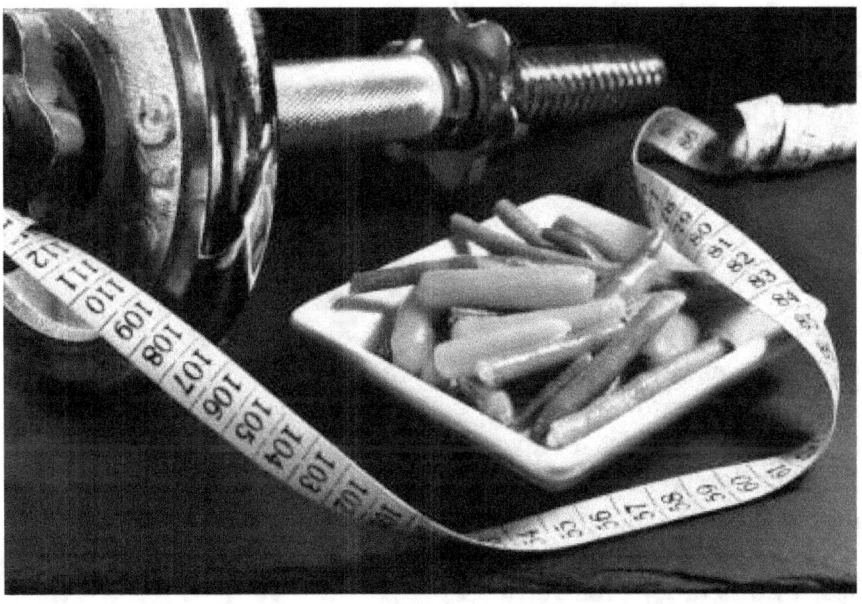

Yes, there is the traditional method of helping to bulk up and get stronger, and that involves eating a diet that is really high in animal fats and animal products. This is one way to do things, but it does make it more likely that the individual is going to deal with things like high blood pressure and high levels of cholesterol due to some of the unhealthy fats and other ingredients that are fond of some of those animal products.

With the vegan diet, we are able to cut out all of that bad stuff, and still give the bodybuilder all of the nutrients and more that they need to do a great job with all of this. We are able to create some of the best results possible, even though we are switching over to a diet plan that is based on plants rather than one that is based on meats and animal products instead. Let's dive in a bit here and learn more about how we can make this work for some of our needs as well.

Contrary to some of the beliefs that are out there, it is possible for bodybuilders to go meat-free and still achieve all of their fitness goals. There is actually a lot of science out there that shows us how we are able to follow this kind of diet and actually achieve some of our goals much faster than before. Although a lot of people in the mainstream fitness community believe that bodybuilders have to consume a huge amount of the animal proteins in order to bulk up and see any results, there are a lot of vegan bodybuilders out there. And many of them have been able to build up their own sexy and strong physiques while focusing on the foods that are only based on plants.

For someone who is brand new to the whole idea of the vegan diet, it is easy to think that all that you need to do here is to cut out the cheese and the eggs in favor of some of the cherished snack foods instead. However, this style of dieting is going to add more flab to the body compared to the muscle tone that you are looking for. To help you to see some more bulk when it comes to veganism, you must make sure that you are going on a whole and healthy diet that will provide the body with all of the nutrients and more that it needs to survive.

Crafting a diet for bodybuilding that is vegan is so important. It is a bit of a challenge though, and you need to have a lot of attention to detail, motivation, and knowledge about the diet plan to start with. Some of the basics and the guidelines that we need to follow in order to stick with the right nutrition for vegan bodybuilding will include:

1. Get the right calories

When you are going on this kind of diet and you plan to be a bodybuilder, then you have to take in the right number of calories. The average vegan diet is going to be lower in calories than some of the conventional diets, so you need to really monitor your levels. If you do not take in enough calories, it is possible that your body is going to enter into a more catabolic state. The larger this deficit, the larger the problem is going to be. To get to your peak performance, you should go for 15 to 20 calories for each pound of bodyweight and then make some adjustments based on the noticeable losses and gains that you see in the gym.

2. Get the protein

While most of us need less protein than we think, it is still important for us to go through and keep our levels of protein levels at a good place, especially if we are doing bodybuilding. As long as you are keeping track of your protein levels and you know which foods are going to have the best protein while still being a part of the vegan diet, then you are going to be just fine.

3. Try some flax seed powder

In addition to the protein, another thing that you need to get in abundant amounts in your diet is lots of omega-3 fatty acids. And since you are not able to have fish on this kind of diet plan, going with the flax seed powder is going to be a good option. This is a good fiber profile and it is going to be a bit easier on the digestive system compared to flaxseed oil. It is going to give you the results that you want if you take it right when you wake up, right after you do some of the training, and right before you go to bed.

4. Take some Vegan BCAA

This is going to be a good option because it will protect your muscles from some of the catabolic effects that happen with a low-calorie diet and can be what you need to gain some more mass. In fact, according to one study that was done in 2010 and published in Med Science Sports Exercise, the BCAA is going to be able to help reduce the amount of soreness that you feel in the muscles when you are done training. For bodybuilding kinds of benefits, you should take some with your breakfast, some before and after training and some before you go to bed.

5. Swap in some quinoa instead of rice.

You will find that rice is going to be one of the staples of this kind of diet plan, which means that it is going to be a really effective method to boost your nutritional intake and protein and when you swap it out for some quinoa, these get even better. Quinoa is going to offer a higher quality of protein and it is more of a complete source compared to brown rice. It also has a lot more of the nutrients that you need to fuel yourself after a workout. It even tastes and feels similar to what we are used to with brown rice so it is not going to feel weird at all.

6. Choose some of the healthier drinks

Just because you are on the vegan diet doesn't mean that you have to spend your time filling the body with lots of sugary drinks with lots of calories and sugars and no Nutritional values per serving. You should keep things simple with a combination of protein shakes, water, tea, and coffee, and nothing else. Make sure that during this diet plan, you are staying as hydrated as possible to keep things running smoothly.

7. Look at some of the supplements for bodybuilding that are vegan

No conversations about this kind of diet and the exercise that you plan to do will be complete without us spending some time talking about the supplements. You will find that these nutritional supplements are going to be a requirement for those who want to body build in a competitive manner and it is likely that this is a trend that is going to stick around for some time. There are a number of great supplements that can help out with this, and many of them are going to be considered vegan so you know you are getting the best nutrition.

8. Address any of the deficiencies that will show up before they become damaging.

When you are going on this kind of diet plan, you need to make sure that you are getting all of the nutrients that you need to stay healthy. It is always a good idea to vary all of the foods and meals that you have in any diet plan because this will ensure that you are not going to suffer from a deficiency in any of them. This is especially true when you are taking the vegan diet like a bodybuilder. It also helps to make the diet more enjoyable overall. Some of the most common vegan deficiencies that you need to worry about will include the following:

1. Zinc
2. Calcium
3. Vitamin D
4. Vitamin B12
5. Omega-3 fatty acids
6. Iodine
7. Iron
8. Calories
9. Protein

If there is any time that you feel your body is starting to get low on one or more of these, then it is time to make some adjustments to your eating plan to make sure that you are able to get back on track. Going with a supplement can be a good option here as well.

As you can see, even bodybuilders are able to go through and follow the vegan diet for some of their needs as well. They may need to go through and create a few different options to ensure that they are getting the best results possible, but it is going to make it a whole lot easier to get some of the performance results that you want because you are actually feeding your body the healthy and wholesome foods and nutrients that it is looking for. The vegan diet is not necessarily the diet plan that most people think about when it comes to bodybuilding, but it is one of the best to choose to stick with.

Part II
Recipes and Meal Plans to Fuel Your Workouts

Chapter 5: The Meal Plan

It is at this point in the process where we need to take some time to talk about the meal plan. We have already taken a look at some of the basics of this kind of diet plan and what it is able to do for us. Even athletes are able to get a lot of benefits when they choose to work with the vegan diet, and we explored that a bit as well. As an athlete though, you do need to take a few precautions along the way to ensure that you are picking out the right meals, and the right amount of variety to ensure you get the nutrients your body needs.

This is probably one of the hardest parts of the whole diet. This is even truer when you are a beginner or when you are trying to get it to work around some of the more complicated nutrient requirements that athletes will sometimes have. This is why we are going to take some time in this chapter looking at the simple meal plan that you are able to follow in order to really do well on the vegan diet while being an athlete.

This meal plan is simple and easy to follow and you will be able to make it work for your needs in no time. Let's take a look at the simple meal plan that athletes are able to follow when they are ready to be on the vegan meal plan.

Day 1:

Breakfast: Mexican Tofu Skillet
Lunch: Stuffed Hummus Pita Sandwich
Dinner: California Veggie Burger

Day 2:

Breakfast: Rolled oats with chia seeds and berries
Lunch: Curried Tofu Salad
Dinner: BBQ Tempeh

Day 3:

Breakfast: Vegan English Muffin
Lunch: Quinoa with spaghetti sauce and black beans
Dinner: Veggie burger

Day 4:

Breakfast: sweet potato toast with avocado
Lunch: Spinach and pepper salad
Dinner: Sweet Potato, Black Bean, and Quinoa Chili

Day 5:

Breakfast: Ezekiel toast with almond butter and apple
Lunch: Leafy green salad
Dinner: Grain Bowl

Chapter 6: Workout Breakfasts

Blueberry Muffins
Prep time 30 minutes
Serves 8

What's inside:
- Blueberries (1 c.)
- Baking soda (.5 tsp.)
- Flour (2 c.)
- Vanilla (1 tsp.)
- Maple syrup (.5 c)
- Applesauce (.5 c.)
- Milk that is plant-based (.5 c.)

How to make
1. Turn on your oven and heat it up to 375 degrees. While the oven is heating up, bring out a big bowl and mix together the vanilla, maple syrup, applesauce, and milk.
2. When this is done, you can add in the flour and the baking soda, stirring until the batter is nice and smooth.
3. When you get the batter to be smooth, you can slowly add in the blueberries to make sure they get distributed through the batter.
4. Then take out a muffin tin and start adding the butter, filling up eight of the muffin cups until they are ¾ of the way full. Add to the oven.
5. After about 25 minutes, the muffins should be all done. You can take them out of the oven at that time and give them a few minutes to cool down before serving.

Nutritional values per serving
Calories 200
Carbs 45g
Fat 1g
Protein 4g

Banana Bread

Cook time 60 minutes
Serves 8

What's inside:
- Walnut pieces, optional (.25 c.)
- Baking soda (.5 tsp.)
- Cinnamon that is ground (.5 tsp.)
- Flour (1.5 c.)
- Vanilla (1 tsp.)
- Apple cider vinegar (1 Tbsp.)
- Maple syrup (.25 c.)
- Bananas that are ripe (4)

How to make this:
1. To start this recipe, turn on the oven and let it heat up to 350 degrees.
2. While the oven is getting nice and warm, bring out a bowl and use a mixing spoon to mash up your bananas until they are pureed well. stir in the vanilla, apple cider vinegar, and the maple syrup at this time.
3. When this is done, you can stir in your baking soda, cinnamon, and flour. Fold in the pieces of walnuts if you are using them.
4. When all of this is combined into a nice batter, you can pour it into your prepared loaf pan and add it to the oven.
5. This needs to cook for a bit of time. After about 60 minutes or so, the bread should be done.
6. Take it out of the oven at this time and give it around half an hour to cool down before you serve.

Nutritional values per serving
Calories 178
Carbs 40g
Fat 1g
Protein 4g

Pancakes

Total time 30 minutes
Serves 4

What's inside:

- Vanilla (1 tsp.)
- Maple syrup (.25 c)
- Applesauce (.5 c.)
- Milk that is plant-based (1 c.)
- Cinnamon that is ground (.5 tsp.)
- Baking powder (1 tsp.)
- Flour (1 c.)

How to make:

1. For this recipe, bring out a bowl and combine together the cinnamon, baking powder, and flour.
2. When those are well combined, you can stir in the vanilla, maple syrup, applesauce, and the milk. You will want to stir these in until there isn't any more dry flour in there and the batter is nice and smooth.
3. When you are ready, heat up a skillet until it is nice and warm. To make each pancake, there should be eight total, you can add .25 cups of the batter onto the skillet.
4. Let it cook for a few minutes. When some bubbles start to form on the top, it is time to flip this around and cook for a bit longer.
5. Repeat the steps until you have been able to use up all of the batters and then serve.

Nutritional values per serving

Calories 219
Carbs 44g
Fat 2g
Protein 5g

Pecan and Maple Granola

Total time 25 minutes
Serves 4

What's inside:

- Ground cinnamon (.5 tsp.)
- Maple syrup (.25 c)
- Vanilla (1 tsp.)
- Pecan pieces (.25 c.)
- Rolled oats (1.5 c.)

How to make this:

1. Turn on the oven to start this and give it time to heat up to 300 degrees. While the oven is heating up, take out a baking sheet and line it with some parchment paper.
2. Then, take out a big bowl and combine together the cinnamon, vanilla, maple syrup, pecan pieces, and the oats. Stir these until the pecan pieces and the oats are coated all the way through.
3. When those are combined, you can spread this mixture out onto the baking sheet that you prepared ad then make it into an even layer. Add to the oven to bake.
4. After about 20 minutes, with a check on them at ten minutes, the granola should be all done. Take these out of the oven and let them set on the counter to cool down for a bit before serving.

Nutritional values per serving

Calories 220
Carbs 35g
Fat 7g
Protein 5g

Overnight Oatmeal

Serves 2

What's inside:

- Chia seeds (1 Tbsp.)
- Maple syrup (1 Tbsp.)
- Sliced banana (1)
- Pineapple chunks (.5 c.)
- Diced mango (.5 c.)
- Milk that is plant-based (2 c.)
- Rolled oats (2 c.)

How to make:

1. Bring out a big bowl and mix together the chia seeds, maple syrup, banana, pineapple, mango, milk, and oats.
2. When this is done, cover up the bowl and add it to the fridge. This needs to set for at least four hours, though leaving it to sit overnight is usually going to be the best.
3. The next morning you can take this out and serve.

Nutritional values per serving:

Calories 510
Carbs 93g
Fat 12g
Protein 14g

Pumpkin Pie Oatmeal

Total time 35 minutes
Serves 4

What's inside:

- Ground nutmeg (.25 tsp.)
- Ground cloves (.25 tsp.)
- Ground cinnamon (1 tsp.)
- Maple syrup (2 Tbsp.)
- Unsweetened pumpkin puree (1 c.)
- Oats (1 c.)
- Milk that is plant-based (3 c.)

How to make this:

1. Brin gout a pan and heat it up on medium heat. Add the milk inside and then let this come to a boil.
2. When the milk is to a rolling boil, you can reduce the heat down to a low ad then stir in the nutmeg, cloves, cinnamon, maple syrup, oats, and pumpkin puree.
3. When all of those are in the pot, cover it up and let these cook for a bit. You will want to stop and stir it every few minutes to help keep it mixed and to make sure that none of the oatmeal is able to stick to the bottom.
4. After about half an hour, this mixture should be done. Pour it into a few bowls before serving.

Nutritional values per serving

Calories 218
Carbs 38g
Fat 5g
Protein 7g

Peanut Butter and Chocolate Quinoa

Total time 25 minutes
Serves 2

What's inside:

- Peanut powder (1 Tbsp.)
- Cocoa powder (1 Tbsp.)
- Maple syrup (1 Tbsp.)
- Cooked quinoa (2 c.)
- Milk that is based on plants (1 c.)

How to make this:

1. Take the time to cook up the quinoa. You can follow the instructions that are on the back of the box that came with it to make this easier.
2. When that is done, bring out another pan and heat it up. Add the milk inside and bring this to a boil as well.
3. When the milk is at a rolling boil, then it is time to reduce the heat a bit to a low setting before adding in the peanut powder, cocoa powder, maple syrup, and the quinoa.
4. Cook these for a bit without the lid on top. After five minutes, with a constant stream of stirring the whole time, you can serve this mixture nice and warm.

Nutritional values per serving:

Calories 339
Carbs 52g
Fat 8g
Protein 14g

Early Morning Scramble

Total time 30 minutes
Serves 2

What's inside:
- Spinach, fresh (1 c.0 pepper
- Onion powder (.5 tsp.)
- Garlic powder (.5 tsp.)
- Vegetable broth or water (1 Tbsp.)
- Nutritional yeast (2 Tbsp.)
- Diced bell pepper (.5)
- Sliced mushrooms (4 oz)
- Tofu (14 oz.)

How to make this:

1. Start out this recipe by taking out a skillet and heat it on the stove.
2. You can drain out your tofu package and then add it into the skillet, mashing it down with a fork or your mashing spoon.
3. When this is done, we can stir in the pepper, onion powder, garlic powder, broth, nutritional yeast, bell pepper, and mushrooms.
4. When all of those are in the skillet, you can cover up the pan and cook for a bit, making sure to stir a few times as well.
5. After ten minutes, you can uncover the pot and then stir in the spinach. Cook for a few more minutes before you serve this warm.

Nutritional values per serving
Calories 230
Carbs 16g
Fat 10g
Protein 27g

Loaded Breakfast Burrito

Total time 30 minutes
Serves 2

What's inside:

- 6 corn tortillas
- Salsa(.25 c.)
- Onion powder (.5 tsp.)
- Garlic powder (.5 tsp.)
- Nutritional yeast (1 Tbsp.)
- Vegetable broth or water (2 Tbsp.)
- Diced and seeded jalapeno (1)
- Sliced mushrooms (4 oz.)
- Cooked black beans (1 c.)
- Diced potatoes (2)
- Firm tofu (.5 block)

How to make this:

1. The first step is to heat up a skillet on the stove and let it get nice and warm.
2. When that is done you can drain out the tofu that you are using and then place it into that pan, mashing it down with a mixing spoon or your form.
3. After this, take the onion powder, garlic powder, nutritional yeast, broth, jalapeno, mushrooms, black beans, and potatoes and add them into that warm skillet.
4. When the ingredients are all inside, you can reduce the heat to a low setting and then covers up the skillet. Cook until the potatoes are nice and soft and can be pierced using a fork.
5. After ten minutes, this part should be done. You can take the cover off the skillet and add in the salsa to heat up. After ten minutes, those should be done as well.

6. Now it is time to warm up the tortillas. Add to the microwave and heat up for 15 to 30 seconds each until they are soft or warm.
7. Take the skillet from the heat and add about 1/6 of the filling into the middle of your tortilla. Roll these up and serve them nice and warm.

Nutritional values per serving

Calories 535
Carbs 95g
Fat 8g
Protein 29g

Sweet Potato Skillet

Total time 30 minutes
Serves 4

What's inside:

- Pepper
- Chili powder (.5 tsp.)
- Ground cumin (.5 tp.)
- Vegetable broth (1 c.)
- Diced sweet onion (1)
- Diced bell pepper (1)
- Sliced mushrooms (8 oz.)
- Diced sweet potatoes (4)

How to make this:
1. Bring out a skillet and give it some time to heat up on the stove.
2. Once you have the time to get the skillet nice and hot, add in the pepper, chili powder, cumin, garlic powder, broth, onion, bell pepper, mushrooms, and sweet potatoes in as well.
3. Cover up the skillet and then let this cook for a bit until the sweet potatoes are all done and we can pierce them easily with a fork.
4. This will all take about ten minutes. When that time is up, take the cover off the skillet and give it a stir. Add in a bit of the broth if needed to get the ingredients to not be stuck on the bottom.
5. Cook without the cover for another five minutes before serving this dish nice and warm.

Nutritional values per serving
Calories 158
Carbs 34g
Fat 1g
Protein 6g

Vegan Omelet

Prep time 30 minutes
Serves 2

What's inside:

- Nutritional yeast (4 Tbsp.)
- Minced garlic cloves (4)
- Hummus (4 Tbsp.)
- Silken tofu (10 oz.)
- Arrowroot powder (2 tsp.)
- Paprika (.5 tsp.)
- Pepper
- Salt

For the filling:

- Vegetables of choice (2 c.)
- *For the toppings*
- Vegan parmesan cheese
- Salsa
- Herbs

How to make this:

1. Start this recipe by turning on the oven and heating it up to 375 degrees. While this is heating up, you can prepare the vegetables to mince the garlic and dry off the tofu before putting it all to the side.
2. Then take out a skillet and heat it up. Add in the garlic and the oil and let it cook for just a few minutes.
3. Add this to the blender along with the rest of the ingredients for the omelet. If you need to thin it out a bit you can add a bit of water at a time.

4. Add some more oil to your skillet and then put the vegetables in as well. These need to go for about 5 minutes.
5. When that time is done, take the skillet off the heat and see that it has enough oil so the omelet is not going to stick. Spoon the batter of the omelet into it along with a bit of the cooked vegetables.
6. Put this back on the stove and cook until you see the edges are starting to dry. After five minutes, add to the oven to finish cooking.
7. After 10 minutes or so, the omelet should be golden brown and done. You can, during the final few minutes, you can add the vegetables back to the top of the omelet and cook for a bit longer.
8. Remove this out of the oven when the time is done and then fold it over with a spatula before serving.

Nutritional values per serving

Calories 232
Carbs 22g
Fat 7.8g
Protein 22g

Chapter 7: Sauces and Dips

BBQ Sauce

Prep time 5 minutes
Serves 12

What's inside:

Tomato sauce, sweet (18 oz.)
Maple syrup (2 Tbsp.)
Apple cider vinegar (1 Tbsp.)
Soy sauce, low in sodium (1.5 Tbsp.)
Chili flakes (1 tsp.)
Sweet paprika (.5 Tbsp.)
Smoked paprika (.5 Tbsp)
Dried oregano (.5 tsp)
Liquid smoke (.5 tsp.)

How to make this:

1. To start this recipe, bring out a bowl and then make sure that all of the ingredients are thrown into it together.
2. You should do some whisking on this until there are no longer any lumps found inside.
3. When this is done, add to a container for about 60 minutes or so before using, or store in the fridge to use later.

Nutritional values per serving
Calories 12
Carbs 2.3g
Fat 0.1g
Protein 0.4g

Your Own Marinara Sauce

Prep time 40 minutes - Serves 13

What's inside:
- Diced tomatoes (4 big cans)
- Chopped basil (1 c.)
- Olive oil (4 Tbsp.)
- Nutritional yeast (4 Tbsp.)
- Garlic cloves (6)
- Oregano, dried (2 tsp.)
- Maple syrup (1.5 Tbsp.)
- Cayenne pepper (.5 tsp.)
- Salt if you would like

How to make this:
1. To start this recipe, take out a big pot and heat it up. When the pot is warm, add in the oil and warm it up with the minced garlic cloves and cook around.
2. After a minute of cooking the garlic, you can continue on by adding in the tomatoes, oregano, cayenne pepper, and then the maple syrup. Add in the amount of salt that you want.
3. It is time to bring all of this to a simmer. Reduce the heat to a lower setting and then cover up the pot. Simmer these ingredients to cook well.
4. After 25 minutes, this should be nice and warm and it is time to add in the basil and then the nutritional yeast. Stir it around and add in some more of the salt and the water if you would like.
5. Store away to use on a dish in the future or add it to your favorite dish.

Nutritional values per serving
Calories 65
Carbs 5g
Fat 4g
Protein 1.5g

Taco Salsa

Prep time 10 minutes
Serves 6

What's inside:

- Pepper and salt to your taste
- Lime (1)
- Chopped cilantro (2 Tbsp.)
- Red onion (.5)
- Jalapeno (1)
- Firm tomatoes (4)

How to make this:

1. Start off by skinning and then seeding your tomatoes. We can then take the jalapeno and remove the stem and the seeds.
2. Then it is time to cut both of these, the jalapeno and the tomatoes, and dice into some fine pieces before adding to a bowl.
3. Now it is time to chop up both your red onion and your cilantro before adding into a bowl. And then juice your lime and add all of that juice into your bowl as well.
4. You can now mix the ingredients and then season with some pepper and salt. Let it marinate together for about 60 minutes before serving.

Nutritional values per serving

Calories 30
Carbs 6.1g
Fat 0.3g
Protein 0.8g

Apple Sauce

Prep time 40 minutes - Serves 4

What's inside:
- Lemon juice (1 Tbsp.)
- Cinnamon (.5 tsp.)
- Salt (1 pinch)
- Water (.5 c.)
- Peeled and quartered red delicious apples (4)
- Peeled and quartered Jazz apples (4)

How to make this:

1. Take the apples and add them to some colder water. This needs to happen for at least 5 minutes or so.
2. When that time is done, we can take the apples out of our water and then slice them all up into quarters.
3. Add these slices into a pan and then cook them with a bit of water and some salt.
4. Stir this often so that it does not burn, and bring it to a simmer right after you notice it is cooking.
5. When ten minutes of cooking is done, you can mash up the apples while they are still in the simmering mode because this will create the sauce.
6. Continue to strand do some mashing in this manner until you have applesauce that is chunky. This will take us around 20 minutes to accomplish.
7. Add in the lemon juice and cinnamon at this point and allow it some time to cool down.
8. If you would like to have it be a bit smoother, you can add to the blender to make it that way before serving.

Nutritional values per serving
Calories 202
Carbs 50.5g
Fat 0g
Protein 0g

Vegan Mayo

Prep time 10 minutes
Serves 6

What's inside:

- Garlic cloves (1)
- MCT oil (1 c.)
- Lemon juice (1 tsp.)
- Almond milk (.5 c.)
- Agave nectar (1 tsp.)
- Rice vinegar (1 tsp.)
- Ground mustard (.5 tsp.)
- Onion powder (1 tsp.)
- Chili powder (1 tsp.)
- Paprika powder (1 tsp.)
- Garlic clove (1)

How to make this:

1. Take out a blender and add in all of the almond milk, mustard, rice vinegar, agave nectar, onion powder, chili powder, paprika, and garlic. Blend to make smooth.
2. Slowly add in the MCT oil to this and blend to make the almond milk and the oil come together well.
3. When you notice that this mixture is starting to get a bit thicker, you can add in some of the lemon juice. Then store this into a glass jar that is sealable before serving.

Nutritional values

Calories 344
Carbs 1.3g
Fat 38g
Protein 0g

Easy Enchilada Sauce

Prep time 10 minutes - Serves 13
What's inside:
- MCT oil (1.5 Tbsp.)
- Chili powder (.5 Tbsp.)
- Whole wheat flour (.5 Tbsp.)
- Ground cumin (.5 tsp)
- Dried or fresh oregano (.25 tsp.)
- Salt (.25 tsp.)
- Minced garlic clove (1)
- Tomato paste of choice (1 Tbsp.)
- Vegetable broth (1 c.)
- Apple cider vinegar (.5 tsp.)
- Pepper (.5 tsp.)

How to make this:
1. Take out a pan and let it heat up on the stove. Wen that is warmed up, you can throw in the minced garlic and the MCT oil and cook these around for 60 seconds or so.
2. Then it is time to bring out a bowl and mix together the flour along with all of the dry spices. Pour the dry mixture into the saucepan.
3. When that is done, stir in the tomato paste and then slowly pour in your vegetable broth at the same time, stirring to make sure that it is all going to come in as we want.
4. When this is thoroughly mixed together well, we can increase the heat a bit and let this simmer so the sauce has the time to thicken.
5. After three minutes of cooking that, we can take the pan from the heat that we are using and add in the pepper and the vinegar before storing or serving.

Nutritional values per serving
Calories 18
Carbs 0.6g - Fat 1.6g - Protein 0.1g

Chapter 8: Easy Lunch Recipes

BBQ Sliders

Total time 30 minutes - Serves 6

What's inside:
- Tomatoes, pickles, onions for topping
- Asian style slaw for topping
- Slider buns (6)
- Onion powder (1 tsp.)
- Garlic powder (1 tsp.)
- BBQ sauce (.5 c.)
- Green jackfruit (2 cans)

How to make this:

1. Bring out a big bowl and use a fork or your own potato masher to help get the jackfruit mashed to a shredded type of consistency.
2. Heat up a stockpot and add in the onion powder, garlic powder, BBQ sauce, and shredded jackfruit.
3. Stir this around and cover the pot. After 10 minutes, then you can take the lid off.
4. If you notice that the jackfruit is starting to stick then you can add in a bit of water or vegetable broth to help with this.
5. When the lid is off, you can cook for a few more minutes to heat all the way up.
6. Serve this on some of the slider buns and add on your favorite toppings before serving.

Nutritional values per serving
Calories 188
Carbs 36g
Fat 2g
Protein 7g

Hawaiian Burgers

Total time 30 minutes
Serves 8

What's inside:

- Toppings of your choice
- Buns (8)
- Pineapple sliced into rings (1)
- Onion powder (1 tsp.)
- Garlic powder (1 tsp.)
- Pineapple juice (.25 c.)
- BBQ sauce (.25 c.)
- Oats that are quick-cooking (1 .c)
- Cooked brown rice (2 c.)
- Cooked black beans (3 c.)

How to make this:

1. Turn on the grill at the beginning of this and get it up to medium-high heat.
2. In the meantime, take out a bowl and use a fork to help mash the black beans in. then add in the onion powder, garlic powder, pineapple juice, BBQ sauce, oats, and rice into it.
3. Combine this mixture until it is able to hold its own shape and can be formed into patties.
4. Scoop out about half a cup of this and form into a patty. Repeat to use up the whole mixture and then add these onto the grill.
5. Cook for about 5 minutes on the one side and then flip them over to cook on that side.
6. Add the pineapple rings on the grill at this time and only cook for a few minutes on each side.

7. When this is done, take the pineapple rings and burgers off the grill. Add one pineapple ring and one patty onto each bun.
8. Top with some of the BBQ sauce and some of the favorite toppings you chose before serving.

Nutritional values per serving

Calories 371
Carbs 71g
Fat 3g
Protein 15g

Falafel Burgers

Total time 30 minutes
Serves 8

What's inside:

- Favorite toppings
- Whole-wheat buns or pita pockets
- Ground pepper (.25 tsp.)
- Ground coriander (1 tsp.)
- Ground cumin (1.5 tsp.)
- Onion powder (2 tsp.)
- Garlic powder (2 tsp.)
- Lemon juice (1 Tbsp.)
- Chopped parsley that is fresh (.25 c.)
- Vegetable broth (.25 c.)
- Brown rice that is cooked (2 c.)
- Cooked chickpeas (3 c.)

How to make this:

1. Turn on the oven and let it heat up to 425 degrees. While the oven is heating up you can take out a baking sheet and line with some parchment paper.
2. Now bring out your food processor and combine the pepper, coriander, onion powder, cumin, garlic powder, lemon juice, parsley, broth, rice, and chickpeas.
3. Process these ingredients together for about half a minute. You don't want it to turn into hummus but have it enough so that it forms into patties.
4. When this is done take about half a cup of the mixture and form it into patties. Add onto your prepared baking sheet and then repeat that with the rest of the mixture.
5. Add this to the oven and let it bake. After 15 minutes, take these out of the oven and then flip them around before cooking for another 15 minutes.

6. When this is done, take the patties out of the oven to cool down. Fill up the buns or the pitas with some of your favorite toppings and then add in the burgers to serve.

Nutritional values per serving

Calories 230
Carbs 44g
Total 3g
Protein 10g

Vegan Pizza Bread

Total time 45 minutes
Serves 4

What's inside:

- Garlic powder (.5 tsp.)
- Onion powder (.5 tsp.)
- Nutritional yeast (1 tsp.)
- Marinara (1 c.)
- An unsliced loaf of bread (1)

How to make this:

1. Turn on the oven and heat it up to 375 degrees.
2. While that is warming up, halve the loaf of bread going lengthwise. Ten spread out the marinara on top f each part before sprinkling on the garlic powder, onion powder, and nutritional yeast.
3. Add the bread onto your prepared baking sheet and then add it into the oven to bake.
4. After 20 minutes, the bread is going to be light and golden brown and you can let it have some time to cool down before serving.

Nutritional values per serving

Calories 230
Carbs 38g
Fat 3g
Protein 13g

Baked Mac and Peas

Total time 60 minutes
Serves 8

What's inside:

- Green peas (2 c.)
- Anytime vegan cheese sauce (1 recipe)
- Macaroni pasta (16 oz.)

How to make this:

1. Turn on the oven and give it time to heat up to 400 degrees.
2. While the oven is getting nice and warm, bring out a big stockpot with some water and use it to cook the pasta until it is al dente. Drain out the pasta and the water when it is done.
3. Then bring out a big baking dish and add the cooked pasta along with the peas and the sauce, making sure to mix well. Add into the oven to bake.
4. After 30 minutes the dish should be a nice golden brown and this is the sign that it is done and ready to take out.
5. Bring it out of the oven and let it cool down before you serve.

Nutritional values per serving

Calories 209
Carbs 42g
Fat 3g
Protein 12g

Sweet Potato Casserole

Total time 45 minutes
Serves 6

What's inside:

- Dried rosemary (1 tsp.)
- Dried thyme (1 tsp.)
- Dried sage (1 Tbsp.)
- Vegetable broth (.5 c.)
- Cooked sweet potatoes (8)

How to make this:

1. Turn on the oven and let it heat up to 375 degrees.
2. While the oven is getting nice and warm, remove and throw out the skins from your sweet potatoes and then add the potatoes into your baking dish.
3. Mash these up with a potato masher or a fork and then stir in the rosemary, sage, thyme, and broth.
4. Add this into the oven and give it some time to bake. After 30 minutes, the sweet potatoes should be done and you can serve warm.

Nutritional values per serving:

Calories 154
Carbs 35g
Fat 0g
Protein 3g

Sunday Roast

Total Time 4 to 6 hours
Serves 8

What's inside:

- Pepper (1 tsp.)
- Garlic powder (1 tsp.)
- Onion powder (1 tsp.)
- Vegetable broth (4 c.)
- Sliced mushrooms (8 oz.)
- Green beans (12 oz.)
- Sweet onion cubed (3)
- Sliced carrots (6)
- Cubed white potatoes (6)

How to make this:

1. When you are ready, take out your slow cooker and get it all set up and ready to go.
2. Then add the pepper, garlic powder, onion powder, broth, mushrooms, green beans, onions, carrots, and potatoes inside. Stir these together well to get the spices to mix in.
3. Add the lid on top and then cook this for four hours on a high setting or six hours on a low setting.
4. Make sure to stir the ingredients together well before serving.

Nutritional values per serving

Calories 190
Carbs 39g
Fat 1g
Protein 8g

Vegetable Stir-Fry

Total time 30 minutes
Serves 4

What's inside:

- Cooked brown rice (4)
- Onion powder (1 tsp.)
- Garlic powder (1 tsp.)
- Water or vegetable broth (.25 c.)
- Green beans (2 c.)
- Green peas (2 c.)

How to make this:

1. To start, bring out a pan and heat it up on the stove. When it is warm, you can add in the onion powder, garlic powder, broth, green beans, and peas. Stir it all around.
2. Cover the pan and then let these cook for a bit. Make sure to stir on a regular basis as well.
3. After 8 minutes you can uncover the pan and add in the brown rice that is already cooked. Let these cook for a bit longer.
4. After 5 minutes, with constant stirring in the meantime, this is going to be ready to serve.

Nutritional values per serving

Calories 233
Carbs 48g
Fat 2g
Protein 8g

Vegetable Spring Rolls with Sauce

Total time 30 minutes
Serves 2

What's inside:

- *Dipping sauce*
- red pepper flakes (.5 tsp.)
- garlic powder (.5 tsp.)
- onion powder (.5 tsp.)
- rice vinegar (1 Tbsp.)
- maple syrup (1 Tbsp.)
- peanut powder (2 Tbsp.)

for the spring rolls:

- Brown rice, cooked (1.5 c.)
- Lettuce leaves (6)
- Rice paper wraps (6)
- Fresh basil (1 bunch)
- Fresh mint (1 bunch)
- Fresh cilantro (1 bunch)
- Shredded carrots (1 c.)

How to make this:

1. We can start with the dipping sauce. To do this, we can take out a pan and heat it up.
2. Add in the red pepper flakes, garlic powder onion powder, rice vinegar, maple syrup, and peanut powder.
3. Cook these in the pan for about 10 minutes, making sure to stir on occasion. After the ten minutes, take off the heat and set to the side to cool down a bit.
4. Bring out a shallow bowl or a pan and pour in a bit of water that is warm. Dip a rice paper wrap into the bowl for about ten seconds.

5. Add to a cutting board or another smooth surface. Then lay a lettuce leaf down flat on the rice paper and add .25 cup of the prepared brown rice to it.
6. Top with some of the shredded carrots and a few leaves of each the basil, mint, and cilantro.
7. Wrap the sides of the rice paper right in the center and then rolls up the wrap from the bottom to the top to make the roll tight. Repeat for the rest of your spring rolls.
8. Serve this with the sauce in a bowl on the side and enjoy it.

Nutritional values per serving

Calories 263
Carbs 46g
Fat 3g
Protein 11g

Orange Tofu Bowl

Total Time 40 minutes
Serves 4

What's inside:

For the tofu:
- Cubed tofu (14 oz)
- Ground pepper (.5 tsp.)
- Onion powder (1 tsp.)
- Garlic powder (1 tsp.)
- Flour (.25 c.)

For the orange glaze:

- Onion powder (.5 tsp.)
- Garlic powder (.5 tsp.)
- Maple syrup (1 Tbsp.)
- Rice vinegar (1 Tbsp.)
- Cornstarch (1 Tbsp.)
- Orange juice (.5 c.)

For the bowl:

- Brown rice, cooked (6 c.)

How to make this:

1. We are going to start by making the tofu part. Start by heating up the oven so that it can reach 400 degrees. While the oven is heating up, line a baking sheet with some parchment paper.
2. In the meantime, take out a bowl and whisk together the pepper, onion powder, garlic powder, and flour. Toss the tofu here and toss to cover completely.

3. Add this to the baking sheet and into the oven to bake for a bit. After 20 minutes turn it around and bake for another 20 minutes before bringing out.
4. Then it is time to make the orange glaze. While your tofu is in the oven, bring out a pan and combine the onion powder, garlic powder, maple syrup, rice vinegar, cornstarch and orange juice inside.
5. Bring this to a boil and then when it reaches that, reduce the heat and simmer for a bit.
6. After ten minutes, take the glaze off the heat and set it to the side.
7. Now it is time to make the bowl. Take the tofu out of the oven and mix it nicely and gently with the orange glaze.
8. When you are ready to serve, put 1.5 cups of the brown rice into a bowl and then top with about $1/4^{th}$ of the orange glaze and tofu here. Serve warm.

Nutritional values per serving

Calories 380
Carbs 65g
Fat 8g
Protein 15g

Mango Chickpea Curry

Total time 30 minutes
Serves 6

What's inside:

- Ground cinnamon (.25 tsp.)
- Onion powder (1 tsp.)
- Garlic powder (1 tsp.)
- Ground coriander (1 tsp.)
- Curry powder (1 Tbsp.)
- Ground ginger (1 Tbsp.)
- Maple syrup (2 Tbsp.)
- Milk that is plant-based (2 c.)
- Mango chunks (2 c.)
- Cooked chickpeas (3 c.)

How to make this:

1. Take out a big stockpot and heat it up on the oven.
2. In this post, you can add in the cinnamon, onion powder, garlic powder, coriander, ginger, curry powder, maple syrup, milk mango, and the chickpeas.
3. After stirring, you can cover up the pot and let it cook, making sure to stir a few times
4. After 10 minutes, you can take the lid off the pot and let it cook a few more minutes before serving warm.

Nutritional values per serving

Calories 219
Carbs 38g
Fat 4g
Protein 8g

Italian Bean Balls

Total time 30 minutes
Serves 6

What's inside:

- Pepper (.25 tsp.)
- Onion powder (1 tsp.)
- Garlic powder (1 tsp.)
- Italian seasoning (1 Tbsp.)
- Marinara (.25 c.)
- Oats that are quick-cooking (1 c.)
- Brown rice that is cooked (1 c.)
- Red kidney beans that are cooked (1.5 c.)
- Cooked black beans (1.5 c.)

How to make this:

1. Turn on the oven and let it heat up to 400 degrees. While the oven is heating up, you can line a baking sheet with a bit of parchment paper.
2. Takeout a big bowl and add the kidney beans and black beans together. Use a fork to help mash these together well.
3. Now add in the pepper, onion powder, garlic powder, Italian seasoning, marinara, oats, and rice and stir them together well to combine.
4. Scoop out about .25 c of the bean mixture and then work to make this into a ball. Add these balls onto your baking sheet.
5. Make sure to repeat these steps with the rest of the bean mixture, leaving enough space so they are not touching. Add the prepared baking sheet into the oven to bake.
6. After half an hour, these balls should be browned and heated all the way through. When this happens, take the balls out of the oven and let them cool before serving with a salad or some vegetables.

Nutritional values per serving

Calories 144
Carbs 26g
Fat 2g
Protein 6g

Crispy Chicken Salad

Prep time 20 minutes
Serves 2

What's inside:

- Vegan mayo (2 Tbsp.)
- Vegan crispy chicken (300 g)
- Sliced tomato (.5)
- Sliced lettuce (.25)

How to make this:

1. To start this recipe, turn on the oven and let it heat up to 350 degrees. When that is all warmed up, add the vegan chicken to the oven and let it cook for a bit.
2. After 15 minutes, the chicken should be done and you can set it to the side to cool down.
3. While the chicken is cooking or cooling down, you can take the tomato and lettuce and chop it up.
4. When it is all done you can add the vegetables to a bowl with the chicken and stir together with the mayo before serving.

Nutritional values per serving

Calories 305
Carbs 17g
Fat 15g
Protein 20g

Arugula and Lentil Salad

Prep time 12 minutes
Serves 2

What's inside:

- Pepper
- Salt
- Balsamic vinegar (2 Tbsp.)
- Arugula (1 handful)
- Cooked brown lentils (1 c.)
- Whole wheat bread (3 slices)
- Sun-dried tomatoes in oil (5)
- Jalapeno (1)
- Olive oil (3 Tbsp.)
- Onion (1)
- Cashews (.75 c.)

How to make this:

1. You can start this recipe by roasting the cashew nuts in a pan for about 3 minutes with the help of a bit of oil. When you are done with these, add them into a big salad bowl for now.
2. Then it is time to dice up the onion and fry for a few minutes, usually around three, with another bit of the oil.
3. As your onion is frying, it is time to chop up the tomatoes and chili and add them to a pan to fry for a bit longer. You can then take these when they are done and add them to the bowl with the cashews.
4. You can then take the bread and chop it into some croutons before frying up in the rest of the oil to make it nice and crunchy. When those are done, add them to the salad bowl as well.
5. Take the arugula and the lentils and add them to this bowl. You need to mix the ingredients well together and

season with some salt, vinegar, and pepper. Serve right away.

Nutritional values per serving

Calories 663
Carbs 64g
Fat 41g
Protein 25g

Quinoa and Vegetables

Prep time 25 minutes - Serves 3

What's inside:
- Basil or parsley
- Green onions (4)
- Corn (1.5 c.)
- Orange bell pepper (1)
- Roma tomatoes (3)
- Garbanzo beans (15 oz.)
- Uncooked white quinoa (1 c.)

For the dressing:
- Olive oil (1 Tbsp.)
- Basil (1.5 tsp.)
- Lemon juice (2 Tbsp.)

How to make this:

1. To start this recipe, you can bring out the quinoa and then follow the directions on the package in order to cook it all up.
2. While your quinoa is cooking, you can whisk together the ingredients that you are using for the dressing and then set to the side.
3. Now we can chop up the tomatoes, pepper, and onions. You can also rinse out and drain the garbanzo beans.
4. Pop your quinoa when it is done into a big bowl and then top with the ingredients for the salad. Pour the dressing on top and stir around to combine well before serving.

Nutritional values:
Calories 488
Carbs 76g
Fat 12g
Protein 18g

Chickpea Sunflower Sandwich

Prep time 20 minutes
Serves 2

What's inside:

For the sandwich:

- Lettuce, tomato, onion, and avocado for toppings
- Rustic bread (4 pieces)
- Pinch of salt and pepper
- Chopped dill (2 Tbsp.)
- Chopped red onion (.25 c.)
- Dijon mustard (.5 tsp.)
- Vegan mayo (3 Tbsp.)
- Sunflower seeds (.25 c.)
- Chickpeas (15 oz.)

Garlic herb sauce:

- Almond milk
- Minced garlic cloves (2)
- Dried dill (1 tsp.)
- Half of a lemon juiced
- Hummus (.25 c.)

How to make this:

1. Mix together all of the ingredients that you will use for the garlic and herb sauce and then set it to the side.
2. You can then add your chickpeas to a bowl and mash it up with a fork for the right texture. Then add in the pepper, salt, dill, red onion, maple syrup, mayo mustard, and sunflower seeds to the mix. Adjust the seasonings to help the taste.

3. You can then take the time to toast the bread and the other toppings of the sandwich such as the lettuce, onion, and tomato.
4. Scoop a good amount of this filling and add to the bread. Add with some of the sauce and toppings that you want and then add on the other two slices of bread before serving.

Chickpea and Lentil Bowl

Prep time 45 minutes - Serves 4

What's inside:
- Salt (1 tsp.)
- Curry powder (.5 tsp.)
- Garam Masala seasoning (2 tsp.)
- Drained chickpeas (15 oz.)
- Diced Roma tomatoes (2)
- Water (1 c.)
- Vegetable broth (2 c.)
- Vegan milk (1 c.)
- Dried red lentils (1.5 c.)
- Diced onion (.5 c.)
- Chopped carrots (2)

How to make this:
1. Take the time to fill up a pan and add in some water. Let it get to boiling and then add in the carrots. After five minutes or so of cooking, drain out the water and set the carrots to the side.
2. While your carrots are boiling, you can heat up a bit of oil in a pan and then add in the onion. Cook for a bit so that the onion can become translucent.
3. In another pan, add in the chickpeas, carrots, milk, water, broth, lentils, and onions together. Season with the spices as well.
4. Bring this to a boil and when it reaches that point, you can reduce the heat a bit and let these ingredients simmer together.
5. After 20 minutes, you can take the whole skillet from the heat and serve it warm.

Nutritional values per serving:
Calories 470
Carbs 79g - Fat 5g - Protein 32g

Vegan Chicken, Tomato and Lettuce Sandwich

Prep time 20 minutes
Serves 2

What's inside:

- Vegan mayo to serve
- Tomato slices (4)
- Lettuce leaves (2)
- Chicken bites, crispy (8)
- Slices of bread (4)

How to make this:

1. Start this recipe by turning on the oven and giving it time to heat up to 350 degrees. Add the vegan chicken to a baking pan and add to the oven to bake.
2. After 15 minutes, the chicken should be done. While those are cooking, you can take the time to slice the tomato and pull off the lettuce leaves that you need.
3. Add some butter and mayo to your slices of bread. Then add on the cooked nuggets to the sandwich and enjoy it when ready.

Nutritional values per serving

Calories 461
Carbs 20g
Fat24g
Protein 17g

Tempeh and Carrot Salad

Prep time 20 minutes
Serves 4

What's inside:

- Liquid smoke (.25 tsp.)
- Sliced tempeh (8 oz.)
- Pepper
- Salt
- Cayenne (2 pinches)
- Parsley (.5 c.)
- Maple syrup (1 Tbsp.)
- Lemon juice (.25 c.)
- Tahini (2 Tbsp.)
- Pepper (.25 tsp.)
- Turmeric powder (.25 tsp.)
- Curry powder (1 Tbsp.)
- Diced onion (1)
- Shredded carrots (4 c.)
- Raw walnuts (1 Tbsp.)
- Soy sauce (2 tsp.)
- Olive oil (1 tsp.)
- Maple syrup (1.5 Tbsp.)

How to make this:

1. Take out a wok or your own frying pan and get it all heated up on the stove. Add in the olive oil. When that is warm, add in the triangles of tempeh along with the soy sauce, maple syrup, and liquid smoke.
2. Cook these for a bit, making sure to flip over the tempeh so that it has time to absorb all of the liquid. Sprinkle on the pieces of walnut and then when this is warm, set it to the side for now.

3. Now it is time to add the spices, onions, raisins, syrup, parsley, soy sauce, lemon juice, and carrots into a bowl. Toss well to coat and add the pepper and salt to taste. Serve with the tempeh on top and enjoy.

Nutritional values per serving

Calories 263
Carbs 27g
Fat 13g
Protein 14g

Kidney Bean and Feta Cheese Salad

Prep time 8 minutes
Serves 2

What's inside:

- Spring onions (1)
- Parsley (.5 c.)
- Vegan feta cheese (.75 c.)
- Cucumber (.5)
- Sweetcorn (.5 can)
- Kidney beans (1 can)

For the dressing:

- Salt
- Pepper
- Honey (1 tsp.)
- Dried oregano (.5 tsp.)
- Cumin (1 tsp.)
- Mustard (1 tsp.)
- Olive oil (2 Tbsp.)
- Juice from half a lime.

How to make this:

1. We want to make sure that we start this by rinsing and draining off our kidney beans and the sweetcorn. Then we can finely chop up the cilantro and the parsley ad dice up our cucumber and green onion.
2. You can then add all the ingredients from above into a big salad bowl. Make sure to crumble the feta cheese on top and then mix it all together well.
3. In a second bowl, we need to take all of the ingredients for the dressing and mix them well in their own bowl.

4. Add this to the salad and toss around to coat before serving.

Nutritional values per serving

Calories 540
Carbs 54g
Fat 28g
Protein 23g

Lentil Salad

Prep time 30 minutes
Serves 5

What's inside:

- Prepared cilantro (.66 c.)
- Roma tomatoes (2)
- Red onion (.5)
- Black beans (15 oz.)
- Red bell pepper (1)
- Brown lentils (1 c.)
- Optional green onions

For the dressing:

- Salt (.25 tsp.)
- Oregano (.5 sp.)
- Cumin (1 tsp.)
- Minced garlic clove (2)
- Dijon mustard (1 tsp.)
- Olive oil (2 Tbsp.)
- Juice from one lime

How to make this:

1. Start this recipe and follow the instructions on the package in order to cook up the lentils. Make sure that they are a bit firm rather than mushy before draining them out.
2. While your lentils are busy cooking, you can work on the dressing. To do this, take all of the ingredients for the dressing and add to a bowl. Take the time to mix them together well.
3. Chop up the cilantro, tomatoes, pepper, and onion at this time. You can then take the prepared lentils and black

beans and all of the chopped vegetables and add to a big bowl.
4. Top it all with the dressing and then serve warm when you are ready.

Nutritional values per serving

Calories 285
Carbs 41g
Fat 6g
Protein 15g

CHAPTER 9: DINNER RECIPES

Vegan Enchiladas

Prep time 50 minutes
Serves 6

What's inside:

For the enchiladas:
- Nutritional yeast (.33 c.)
- Hemp hearts (.5 c.)
- Garbanzo beans (1 can)
- Black bans (1 can)
- Red bell pepper (1)
- Onion (1)
- Tortillas (6)
- Salt
- Smoked paprika (1 tsp.)
- Cumin (2 tsp.)
- Tomatoes, Roma (3)

Sauce:
- Pepper
- Salt
- Onion powder (.25 tsp.)
- Garlic powder (.5 tsp.)
- Chili powder (.5 tsp.)
- Cumin (2 tsp.)
- Olive oil (2 Tbsp.)
- Flour (.25 c.)
- Tomato paste (.25 c.)
- Vegetable broth (3 c.)

How to make this:

1. To get started on this one, we are going to make the sauce. To do this, we can take out a bowl and combine the flour, onion powder, chili powder, garlic powder, and cumin in a bowl.
2. When that is done, heat up a bit of oil in a pan and then add in the spice and flour mixture along with the tomato paste. Cook for a minute, making sure to stir the whole time.
3. After a minute, you can add in the broth and bring it to a boil. Reduce the heat and let this simmer for a bit. That will take around eight minutes.
4. Now we can work on the enchiladas of this. You can turn on the oven to reach 350 degrees. While that is heating up, take the time to dice up your onion and bell pepper.
5. In a pan, you can add a bit of oil along with those prepared onions and peppers for a bit.
6. Rinse off the beans and dice the tomatoes as those are cooking. Then add the beans, hemp hearts, yeast, paprika, cumin and tomatoes to the frying pan.
7. Give all of this a good stir around and then heat for a bit before you set it aside for now.
8. Prepare a baking dish and then cover the bottom with just a bit of the sauce, but do not use it all.
9. Fill each of the tortillas with the bean mixture that we have and then roll them up before adding to the baking dish. Cover these with the remainder of the sauce and then add into the oven.
10. After about 25 minutes, these should be done. Take them out of the oven so they can cool down before adding some of your favorite toppings and serving.

Nutritional values per serving:
Calories 526
Carbs 68g
Fat 19g
Protein 22g

Tex-Mex Tofu with Beans

Prep time 25 minutes
Serves 4

What's inside:

- Pepper and salt to taste
- Chili powder (1 tsp.)
- Paprika (2 tsp.)
- Cumin (2 tsp.)
- Lime juice (1 Tbsp.)
- Minced garlic clove (1)
- Pitted avocado (1)
- Diced onion, purple (1)
- Olive oil (2 Tbsp.)
- Firm tofu (14 oz.)
- Brown rice, dry (1 c.)
- Black beans, dry (1 c.)

How to make this:

1. Take some time to prepare the black beans and the brown rice by following the directions on the package.
2. While those are getting ready, we can slice up the tofu into cubes. Then heat up a bit of oil in a skillet. Add in the onions and then cook to make them nice and soft.
3. After 5 minutes of cooking the onion, you can add in the tofu and cook for a few more minutes, flipping around the cubes on a regular basis.
4. In the meantime, slice the avocado up and then leave on the side for now. Lower the heat a bit and mix in the cumin, garlic, and the prepared black beans.
5. Make sure to stir all of this so that it can be combined and then heat all the way through.

6. After 5 minutes, you can add in the rest of the lime juice and spices. Mix it all the way through and remove the skillet from the heat.
7. Serve this tofu and beans with some of the rice and then garnish with some of the avocados as well.

Nutritional values per serving

Calories 315
Carbs 28g
Fat 17g
Protein 12.7g

Tofu Cacciatore

Prep time 45 minutes
Serves 3

What's inside:

- Drained tofu (14 oz.)
- Olive oil (1 Tbsp.)
- Carrots, matchstick (1 c.)
- Diced onion, sweet (1)
- Diced green bell pepper (1)
- Diced tomatoes (28 oz.)
- Tomato paste (4 oz.)
- Balsamic vinegar (.5 Tbsp.)
- Soy sauce (1 Tbsp.)
- Maple syrup (1 Tbsp.)
- Garlic powder (1 Tbsp.)
- Italian seasoning (1 Tbsp.)
- Pepper and salt to your taste

How to make this:

1. Take the tofu and chop it into the cubes in the size that you would like. Now we can bring out a skillet and heat up some of the oil inside until nice and hot.
2. When that happens, it is time to add the bell peppers, carrots, garlic, and onions. Let these all cook together until they turn translucent.
3. After ten minutes, making sure you stir often to prevent any burning, the mixture is done.
4. When this part is done, combine the Italian seasoning, garlic powder, maple syrup, soy sauce and balsamic vinegar inside of the pan.
5. You want to stir this while adding in the diced tomatoes and the tomato paste. Mix in all of the ingredients until they are combined and then add in the tofu.

6. This is when we need to cover up the pot and turn down the heat just a bit. Allow the mixture some time to simmer so the sauce has some time to thicken.
7. After 20 minutes of this cooking, you can serve this in a bowl with some pepper and salt and then enjoy it.

Nutritional values per serving

Calories 274
Carbs 34g
Fat 9.5g
Protein 13g

Mushroom Stroganoff

Prep time 30 minutes
Servs 4

What's inside:

- Noodles (2 c.)
- Chopped onion (1)
- Vegetable broth (2 c.)
- Almond flour (2 Tbsp.)
- Tamari (1 Tbsp.)
- Tomato paste (1 tsp.)
- Lemon juice (1 tsp.)
- Chopped mushrooms (3 c.)
- Thyme (1 tsp.)
- Raw spinach (3 c.)
- Apple cider vinegar (1 Tbsp.)
- Olive oil (1 Tbsp.)
- Pepper and salt to your tasting
- Diced parsley (2 Tbsp.)

How to make this:

1. Take some time to prepare the noodles by following the instructions on the package.
2. While that is cooking, heat up a bit of olive oil in a skillet until it is nice and warm. When that happens, you can add in the chopped onion and let it cook until soft.
3. After five minutes of cooking the onion, stir in the lemon juice, tomato paste, tamari, vegetable broth, and the flour and cook to heat all the way through.
4. After that three minutes are done, add in the salt, thyme, and mushrooms and cover up the skillet to cook. We want to cook this until we get mushrooms that are nice and tender.

5. When seven more minutes have gone by, we can turn down the heat a bit and add in the vinegar, spinach, and cooked noodles. Season a bit with some pepper and salt.
6. Cover up that skillet a second time and cook a bit longer, another 10 minutes, so that the flavors are able to combine.
7. Serve this right away.

Nutritional values

Calories 200
Carbs 28g
Fat 6.5g
Protein 8g

BBQ Grits and Greens

Prep time 60 minutes
Serves 4

What's inside:

- Salt (1 tsp.)
- Garlic cloves (2)
- Olive oil (2 Tbsp.)
- Diced white onion (.25 c.)
- Grits (1 c.)
- BBQ sauce (.5 c.)
- Chopped collard greens (3 c.)
- Vegetable broth (3 c.)
- Tempeh (14 oz.)

How to make this:

1. To start this recipe, take the time to heat up the oven to 400 degrees. While that is warming up, take out the tempeh and slice it up thinly before adding with the BBQ sauce into a baking dish.
2. Set this aside and give it some time to marinate for as long as needed.
3. Take out a frying pan and heat up just one tablespoon of the oil inside of it. When that is warm, add in the garlic and cook to make nice and fragrant. Add the collard greens and cook until these are dark and wilted.
4. Take your pan off the heat and then cover the BBQ sauce and tempeh with some foil. Place this whole baking dish into the oven and let it bake for a bit.
5. After 15 minutes of baking, we can uncover that pan and let it bake a bit longer, allowing the tempeh to get crispy and brown.
6. After that ten minutes, we can take this out of the oven and set it to the side.

7. While the tempeh is cooking, heat up the rest of the oil in the frying pan and cook the onion until they are brown. Add in the vegetable broth and bring it all to a boil before turning down to low.
8. Whisk in your grits to this simmering broth. Add the rest of the salt and then put the lid on top to cook.
9. Let these ingredients all simmer together for a bit so the grits have time to get creamy and soft. Serve the collard greens and tempeh on the grits and enjoy.

Nutritional values

Calories 394
Carbs 39g
Fat 17.6g
Protein 20g

Easy Burritos

Prep time 50 minutes
Serves 4

What's inside:

- Salt (.5 tsp.)
- Cilantro (1 Tbsp.)
- Salsa (.75 c.)
- Diced avocado (1)
- Tortilla wraps (4)
- Potatoes (2)
- Portobello mushrooms (3)

For the marinade:

- Teriyaki sauce (.25 c.)
- Minced garlic (1 Tbsp.)
- Lime juice (1 Tbsp.)
- Water (.33 c.)

How to make this:

1. Turn on the oven to start this and heat it up to 400 degrees. While the oven is getting nice and warm, you can add some oil onto a sheet pan and then set it to the side.
2. Bring out a bowl and combine together the garlic, teriyaki, lime juice, and water.
3. Slice up the mushrooms so that they are nice and thin and then add these into the other marinade. Allow this to sit for a maximum o three hours.
4. Now it is time to slice up the potatoes to look kind of like French fries. Sprinkle the fries with some salt and then move them over to the prepared sheet pan.

5. Place these fries into the oven and let them bake to become crispy. After half an hour, you can take these out and set to the side.
6. Bring out a frying pan now and heat it up with the mushroom slices and the rest of the marinade liquid as well. cook these until all of the liquid is gone and evaporated.
7. After ten minutes or so, take these off the heat. Start to assemble the tortillas by adding in a big scoop of the mushrooms and a handful of the potato sticks.
8. Top it all with the cilantro, sliced avocados, and salsa before enjoying it.

Nutritional values per serving

Calories 239
Carbs 34g
Fat 9g
Protein 5g

Fajitas

Prep time 30 minutes
Serves 8

What's inside:

- Salt
- Cayenne pepper (.25 tsp.)
- Garlic powder (1 tsp.)
- Chili powder (1 tsp.)
- Lime juice (1 tsp.)
- Tortilla wraps (6)
- Olive oil (2 Tbsp.)
- Sliced portobello mushrooms (3)
- Chopped onion, sweet (1)
- Mashed avocado (1)
- Sliced poblano pepper (1)
- Diced bell pepper, green (1)
- Black beans, dry (1 c.)

How to make this:

1. Take some time to prepare the black beans using the method that you prefer.
2. When this is done, we can heat up the oil inside one of our frying pans until it is hot. Then add in the bell peppers and the poblano peppers along with half the onion. Add a bit of salt to your own tastes.
3. Cook these vegetables so they have time to get browned and are tender. After ten minutes it is time to add in the black beans and cook until all warmed out.
4. This is the time that we need to add in the mushrooms to the skillet and turn down the heat to a low setting. Stir around the ingredients and cook until the mushrooms are about half their size. Then take it off the heat when this is done.

5. Take out a bowl and combine the rest of the onions with the avocado and the rest of the oil. Mix in some lime juice and add some of the other seasonings as needed.
6. Spread the guacamole that we have onto the tortilla and then add in a big spoon of the prepared mushroom mixture. Serve this and enjoy it right away.

Nutritional values per serving

Nutritional values 264
Carbs 28g
Fat 14g
Protein 6.8g

Farro Protein Bowls

Prep time 40 minutes
Serves 2

What's inside:

- Lemon wedges (4)
- Roasted almonds (2 Tbsp.)
- Hummus (.25 c.)
- Mixed greens (2 c.)
- Pepper
- Salt
- Uncooked farro (.5 c.)
- Diced sweet potatoes (1 c.)
- Diced carrots (1 c.)
- Organic cooking oil (2 tsp.)
- Prepared chickpeas (15 oz.)
- Smoky tempeh strips (4 oz.)
- Water (1.25 c.)

How to make this:

1. To start this recipe, we can turn on the oven and let it heat up to 350 degrees. While that is heating up, add the sweet potatoes to a bowl with the carrots, a small bit of oil and the pepper and salt and mix around to coat.
2. Move this prepared mixture to a baking tray, but only have it take up about a third of the tray.
3. Then it is time to work on the chickpeas. Add these to a bowl with a bit of the oil and some salt and pepper to coat. Toss around to combine and then add onto the baking tray as well.
4. You will want to finish up the room on the baking tray with some of the tempeh strips. When all of these are set up, add the sheet to the oven to roast.

5. After half an hour, you can take these out and give them time to cool down. Make sure to flip them around about halfway through the process.
6. While the stuff is cooking in the oven, you can take out a small pan and add the grains of farro, water, and some salt there. Turn it up to a boil, and then reduce to a simmer until it all is soft.
7. After 25 minutes, this will be done and you can divide the farro between two bowls. Remove the tray from the oven at this time and divide it up as well.
8. Top all of this with the almonds, hummus, and lemon wedges.

Nutritional values per serving

Calories 485
Carbs 73g
Fat 15g
Protein 25g

Seitan Wings

Prep time 30 minutes
Serves 4 (each serving has four wings in it)

What's inside:

For the sauce:
- ketchup (1 Tbsp.)
- Lime juice (1 Tbsp.)
- Vegan butter (.5 c.)
- Hot sauce (.5 c.)

Breading:
- Panko breadcrumbs (.5 c.)
- Flour (.5 c.)
- Paprika (.5 Tbsp.)
- Salt
- Oil (2 Tbsp.)
- Soy milk (1 c.)
- Lime juice (1 Tbsp.)

For the seitan:
- Sliced mushrooms (1 c.)
- Chopped onions (.33 c.)
- Minced garlic (1 Tbsp.)
- Olive oil (2 Tbsp.)
- Ground sage (2 tsp.)
- Ground thyme (1.5 tsp.)
- Ground marjoram (1 tsp.)
- Ground rosemary (.75 tsp.)
- Nutmeg (.5 tsp.)
- Pepper (.5 tsp.)
- Salt (1 tsp.)
- Vegetable broth (.5 c.)
- Vital wheat gluten (1 c.)

How to make this:

1. To start this recipe, we need to take the time to heat the oven to 400 degrees. Then we can add the onion, garlic, and mushrooms to a blender to pulse.
2. Add in the oil, salt, and the rest of the spices that are in the section above for the seitan and pulse it a few more times.
3. Add in the broth here and pulse a bit longer to make a nice smooth paste. Then add in the gluten and process to make the whole thing into a kind of dough.
4. Roll out this dough so that it is able to turn into pieces that are shaped like fingers and then flatten them each out.
5. Then it is time for us to work on making the breading. To do this, we just need to take out a bowl and mix together the pepper, salt, paprika, flour, and breadcrumbs together.
6. In a new bowl, mix the lime juice and the soy milk to make our binding for the brad.
7. Dip all of the pieces of seitan into the lime and soy mixture, and then dump into the breadcrumb mixture before adding to the baking tray. Add to the oven when all of the pieces are done.
8. After 20 minutes of cooking, we can take these out to cool down. The last thing to work on is the sauce. To make this, take out a pan and add the hot sauce, ketchup, lime juice, and butter and heat it up.
9. After 5 minutes, you can pour into a little serving bowl and serve the wings inside.

Nutritional values per serving:
Calories 572
Carbs 36g - Fat 32g - Protein 28g

Easy Dinner Tacos

Prep time 40 minutes
Serves 3

What's inside:

- Coconut oil (1 Tbsp.)
- Organic tempeh (8 oz.)
- Taco shells (6)

For the marinade:

- Onion powder (.25 tsp.)
- Garlic powder (.5 tsp.)
- Tamari (1 Tbsp.)
- Veggie broth (3 Tbsp.)

For the teriyaki sauce:
- Liquid smoke (.25 tsp.)
- Corn starch (.5 tsp.)
- Garlic powder (.5 tsp.)
- Apple cider vinegar (1 tsp.)
- Sriracha (1 tsp.)
- Maple syrup (2 Tbsp.)
- Olive oil (1 tsp.)
- Tamari (4 Tbsp)

For the Asian slaw:

- Pepper (.25 tsp.)
- Salt (.25 tsp.)
- Sriracha (1 Tbsp.)
- Dijon mustard (1 Tbsp.)
- Maple syrup (1 Tbsp.)
- Tamari (.5 Tbs.)
- Lime juice (1 Tbsp.)

- Sesame oil (2 Tbs.)
- Apple cider vinegar (.25 c.)
- Chopped scallions (3)
- Grated carrots (1 c.)
- Shredded red cabbage (1 c.)
- Shredded green cabbage (1 c.)

How to make this:

1. To start this recipe, we are going to work on the slaw. Just take out a bowl, put all of the ingredients inside, and then mix it up well.
2. To make the marinade, we just need to find a second bowl, add in all of the ingredients for that part, and mix well. Set to the side for now.
3. The third thing that we need to do here is to work on our teriyaki sauce. To do this, just add the ingredients inside a bowl and then mix it around.
4. Now it is time to work on the tempeh. We can d this by slicing into triangles. Add these to the marinade that we just made and then set to the side for a bit.
5. After 20 minutes, this should be ready. You can take out a skillet and heat it up. Add the tempeh into it and cook for a few minutes on each side to make nice and crispy.
6. Take the tempeh out of the heat, and then dunk it into the teriyaki sauce that we made before. Then add back to the pan to caramelize the tempeh for another half a minute on each side.
7. Take these off the heat and add more of the sauce if you would like. Add to the tacos and serve with the Asian slaw that we made.

Nutritional values per serving:

Calories 550
Carbs 44g - Fat 31g - Protein 22g

Grilled Tofu Steaks

Prep time 25 minutes
Serves 2

What's inside:

- Soy sauce (2 Tbsp.)
- Tofu (1 block)
- Breadcrumbs (.5 c.)
- Maple syrup (1 tsp.)
- Sesame oil (2 tsp.)
  miso paste (2 tsp.)
- Tomato paste (2 tsp.)

How to make this:

1. Take the time to drain off and press the tofu. Your goal is to get rid of as much of the water from it as you can. When that is done, you can cut this into four layers to make the strips.
2. In a small bowl, take the time to mix together the sesame oil, syrup, tomato paste, miso paste, and soy sauce.
3. Add some oil to a grilling tray. While that heats up, you can dip the strips of tofu into the sauce before adding them into the breadcrumbs as well. add these onto the tray when that is all done with as well.
4. Add these to the grill and do about ten minutes of grilling on one side and about 6 minutes on another side to make them nice and browned all over. Serve with a salad to enjoy.

Nutritional values per serving:

Calories 357
Carbs 29g - Fats 14g - Protein 23g

Vegan Hot Dogs

Prep time 15 minutes
Serves 2 (1 serving is 2 hot dogs)

What's inside:

- Condiments and sauces of your choice
- Chopped onion (.5)
- Hot dogs or sausages that are vegan (4)
- Hot dog rolls (4)

How to make:

1. First, we want to turn on the oven and let it heat up to 360 degrees. Then add the vegan hot dogs inside to cook.
2. After 15 minutes, the hot dogs are done and you can take them out of the oven and add to some hot dog rolls.
3. As the sausage is cooking, you can fry up the onions with a bit of oil on high heat. It will take three minutes to soften them up the way that we want, but you can cook a bit longer if you want.
4. Spoon these on top of your hot dogs and then finish off with some of the condiments and sauces that you would like.

Nutritional values per serving

Calories 550
Carbs 62g
Fats 19g
Protein 24g

Sausage and Tomato Pasta

Prep time 20 minutes
Serves 2

- Mushrooms (3)
- Pepper (1)
- Pasta of choice (2 c.)
- Vegan sausages (6)

For the tomato sauce:

- Pepper
- Salt
- Chili flakes (1 tsp.)
- Basil (1 tsp.)
- Tomato puree (1 Tbsp.)
- Chopped tomato (1)

How to make this:

1. Turn on the oven and give it some time to heat up to 260 degrees. Then add the sausages inside and let them cook up. Look at the instructions on the package to see how long they go.
2. Then bring out a pot and add some water to it. Bring this to a boil and then cook up the pasta until it is all done.
3. Then we need a frying pan and we can add up a few tablespoons of oil inside. As this is heating up, you can chop the mushrooms and peppers and then add them to the pan to cook.
4. After five minutes there will be done. Then as these are cooking, you can add all of the ingredients for the sauce into the blender and pulse to make smooth, but not super thin in the process.

5. Add your sauce to the same pan as the vegetables and let it simmer, not getting too hot, for a bit.
6. When the pasta is all done, you can take the pot off the heat and then drain it all out. Add it back to the pan and then top with the sauce and vegetable mix.
7. Take the vegan sausages out of the oven and slice up. Add to the pasta and mix around before serving.

Nutritional values per serving

Calories 426
Carbs 54g
Protein 32g
Fats 9g

Mongolian Seitan

Prep time 30 minutes
Serves 6

What's inside:

For the sauce:

- Coldwater (2 Tbsp.)
- Cornstarch (2 tsp.)
- Coconut or brown sugar (.5 c. and 2 Tbsp.)
- Soy sauce (.5 c.)
- Red pepper flakes (.33 tsp.)
- Chinese five-spice (.33 tsp.)
- Grated garlic (3 cloves)
  grated ginger (.5 tsp.)
- Vegetable oil (2 tsp.)

For the prepared seitan:

- Seitan cubed (1 lb.)
- Vegetable oil (1.5 Tbsp.)

For serving:

- Sliced scallions
- Toasted sesame seeds

How to make this:

1. Start by heating up the oil on medium heat in your pan. When that is warm, you can add in the ginger and the garlic and stir around.
2. About half a minute later, it is time to add in the red pepper flakes and five spices and cook until fragrant as well.

3. Now it is time to add in the sugar and soy sauce and then lower the heat so these ingredients will simmer. Go until the sugar is dissolved.
4. After 5 minutes, whisk together the water and the cornstarch in a small bowl and then add to the pan to cook until the sauce starts to look a bit glossy.
5. Get the heat down to the lowest setting possible and let it simmer nice and slowly until it is time to add in the seitan.
6. To make our seitan, we want to bring out another pan or a skillet and heat up the vegetables. Add in the seitan and cook for a bit so that it gets browned and starts to be crisp around the edges.
7. This is the time where we reduce the heat to low and add some of the sauce to the pan. Make sure to stir around so that the seitan pieces will get nice and coated.
8. When that is done, you can take it off the heat and serve hot with the vegetables of your choice or with some rice.

Nutritional values per serving

Calories 272
Carbs 22g
Fats 10g
Protein 25g

Vegan Burgers

Prep time 15 minutes
Serves 2 (1 serving is 2 burgers)

What's inside:

- Ketchup or relish to your taste
- Sliced tomato (.5)
- Pulled lettuce leaves (.25)
- Vegan burgers of choice (4)
- Burger buns (4)

How to make this:

1. Take the burgers out of their package and heat up the oven so that it reaches 360 degrees. Add the burgers inside and let them cook for a bit.
2. After 20 minutes, the burgers will b done and you can take them out of the oven to cool down.
3. While that happens, you can slice up your tomato and then pull the leaves off the lettuce that you want to use.
4. Add the prepared burgers onto some buns and top with the tomato and lettuce. Add on any of the sauces that you would like to use as well here.

Nutritional values

Calories 700
Carbs 65g
Fats 27g
Protein 44g

Lentil Loaf with BBQ

Prep time 90 minutes
Serves 2 (2 serving is four slices)

What's inside:

For the loaf:

- Corn (.5 c.)
- Chipotle chili spice (.5 tsp.)
- Ground flaxseed (3 Tbsp.)
- Grind coarse cornmeal (.5 c.)
- BBQ (1 c.)
- Water (.25 c.)
- Salt (.25 tsp.)
- Minced garlic (1 Tbsp.)
- Chopped white onion (.5 c.)
- Salt (.5 tsp.)
- Lentils (1 c.)

For the BBQ:

- Liquid smoke (2 tsp.)
- Regular molasses (2 Tbsp.)
- Dark balsamic vinegar (2 Tbsp.)
- Maple syrup (2 Tbsp.)
- Mustard (1 Tbsp. and 1 tsp.)
- Chili powder (1 tsp. and 1 Tbsp.)
- Garlic powder (.5 Tbsp.)
- Salt (.25 tsp.)
- Water (.5 c.)
- Tomato paste (.5 c.)

How to make this:

1. We want to start this one out by making the sauce. All that is needed for this one is to take all of the ingredients and add them to a bowl, mixing around well.
2. Take out a pan and add in just a bit of oil. When that is hot, add in the garlic and the onions and let them cook until soft.
3. Take out your blender here and puree half of the lentils inside. Then add the garlic and onion to the lentils while mixing in .75 cup of the BBQ sauce here.
4. We also want to add in the flaxseed, cornmeal, and chipotle spice here. Give it all a nice stir until it is thick and sticky before adding in the corn.
5. This is the time to add some baking paper to a metal loaf. Leave a bit over the edges so that it is easier to pull out later.
6. Pour your mixture into the prepared pan and then set it to the side for about twenty minutes or so. At that time, let the oven heat up to 360 degrees for a bit.
7. When you are ready, you can spread the rest of the sauce over your loaf and then add it to the oven. We want to cook until this is nice and firm.
8. After an hour of cooking, take the loaf out of the oven and give it some time to cool down. Then you can take it out of the tin and slice up before serving.

Nutritional values

Calories 520
Carbs 120g
Fats 7g
Protein 23g

Lentil Ragu

Prep time 50 minutes
Serves 4

What's inside:

- Courgettes sliced into noodles (2)
- Balsamic vinegar (2 Tbsp.)
- Dried oregano (1 tsp.)
- Vegetable bouillon (1 liter)
- Passata (1 package)
  dried red lentils (500 grams)
- Quartered button mushrooms (.5 c.)
- Chopped onion (2)
- Chopped garlic cloves (40
  chopped carrots (2)
- Chopped celery sticks (3)
- Rapeseed oil (2 Tbsp.)

How to make this:

1. Take out a pan and heat up two tablespoons of the oil. When this is nice and warm, add the onions, garlic, celery, and carrots inside.
2. Fry these for about 5 minutes on high heat until they start to get soft. Then add in the mushrooms and fry a bit longer.
3. After two minutes of those frying, it is time to add in the balsamic vinegar, oregano, passata, bouillon, and lentils.
4. Cover up the pan here and let it simmer until the lentils are nice and tender, which can take around half an hour. Check on it occasionally to stir and make sure that nothing is sticking. If you need to, add just a bit of water to the mixture.

5. Then we can heat up the rest of the oil in another pan and add in the sliced up courgette. Fry this to make it warm and soft.
6. Serve the Ragu that we made with the courgette and enjoy it.

Nutritional values per serving

Calories 578
Carbs 87g
Fat 7g
Protein 18g

Seitan and Black Bean Stir Fry

Prep time 15 minutes
Serves 2

What's inside:

For the sauce:

- Chinese five-spice powder (1 tsp.)
- Soy sauce (2 Tbsp.)
- Garlic cloves (3)
- Brown sugar (75g)
- Black beans (400g)
- Chopped red chili (1)
- Peanut butter (1 Tbsp.)
- Rice vinegar (2 Tbsp.)

For the stir fry:

- Cooked noodles or rice
- Sliced spring onions (2)
- Chopped pak choi (300 grams)
- Sliced red pepper (1)
- Vegetable oil (3 Tbsp.)
- Corn flour (1 Tbsp.)
- Marinated seitan pieces (350 grams)

How to make this:

1. Take some time to cook up the rice or the rice noodles that you want to use. You can just follow the instructions on the package to get this one done.
2. While the noodles or rice are cooking, you can work on the sauce. You can add half the black beans with the rest of the sauce ingredients into a blender.

3. Blend these together until they are smooth. Add into a pan and cook up for about five minutes inside.
4. As the sauce is getting nice and warm, you can add the seitan with the cornflour. Take out a big frying pan and add in a bit of oil. Then add in the seitan and let it cook until it is golden brown in color.
5. After 5 minutes, you can take the seitan off the heat. Add the spring onion, pak choi, and peppers to the pan with a bit of the oil and fry for a few more minutes before adding the seitan back in.
6. Stir it all together for a minute and then serve warm.

Nutritional values per serving

Calories 660
Carbs 74g
Fat 16 g
Protein 44g

Vegan Sausage Rolls

Prep time 1 hour
Serves 5

What's inside:

- Chopped chestnuts (30 gramso Dijon mustard (2 tsp.)
- Brown rice miso (1 Tbsp.)
- Chopped sage leaves (1 Tbsp.)
- Chopped leeks (2)
- Olive oil (3 Tbsp.)
- Chestnut mushrooms (250 grams)
- Dairy-free milk of choice to glaze
- Plain flour to use for dusting
- Pastry puff sheet (1)
- White breadcrumbs (70 gramso

How to make this:

1. You can start this recipe by adding the mushrooms into a blender and then pulse the ingredients until they are chopped up well.
2. Then we can heat up about half of our oil into a frying pan and when it is warm, add the leeks to cook to make them golden brown and soft.
3. After 15 minutes, these leeks should be done and you can take them off the heat and set to the side.
4. Add in the remainder of your oil to the pan and fry up the mushrooms that you blended. This will take about 10 minutes and then you can add in the miso, mustard, sage, and garlic, frying a bit longer.
5. Turn on the oven here and heat it up to 400 degrees. As the oven is heating up, add the mushroom mixture and the leeks into a bowl together along with the breadcrumbs and the chestnuts.

6. Make sure to season this well and mix it to get it into a stuffing mixture. Then roll out the pastry on a surface that has been floured and then arrange this mixture right in the middle of the pastry for now.
7. When that is done, you can roll up the pastry so that it goes around the filling, sealing it up at the seam with the help of a fork. Cut into 10 rolls and add to a prepared baking tray.
8. Brush each piece of this with some milk and then add to the oven to bake. After 25 minutes, they should be a deep golden brown color and you can take them out.
9. Sprinkle on a few sesame seeds before serving.

Nutritional values per serving

Calories 652
Carbs 54g
Fat 40g
Protein 14g

Spicy Rice in One Pan

Prep time 20 minutes
Serves 4

What's inside:

- Spinach (175 grams)
- Handful of raisins
- Chickpeas (400 grams)
- Vegetable stock (450 ml)
- Rinsed basmati rice (250 grams)
- Curry paste (2 Tbsp.)
- Crushed garlic cloves (2)
- Sunflower oil (1 Tbsp.)
- Serve with natural oil.

How to make this:

1. Take out a large pan and heat up a bit of oil inside. When it gets nice and warm, then you can go through and add in the curry paste and garlic and let these heat up.
2. After a minute, you can add in the pepper, salt, chickpeas, raisins, vegetable stock, and rice. Stir these together well.
3. Reduce the heat a bit and then cover up the pan, letting it heat up and get warm and cooked through.
4. After about 15 minutes, all of the liquid should be gone and your rice should be tender. Right at the end of the cooking process, add in the cashew nuts and spinach.
5. Serve when it is all done.

Nutritional values per serving

Calories 380
Carbs 66g
Fat 9g
Protein 12g

Vegan Banh Mi

Prep time 15 minutes
Serves 4

What's inside:

- Coriander (.5 pack)
- Cooked tempeh (175g)
- Hummus (100 gramso
French baguette (1)
- Golden caster sugar (1 tsp.)
- White wine vinegar (3 Tbsp.)
- Shredded raw veggies (150 grams)
- Hot sauce for serving
- Mint (.5 pack)

How to make this:

1. Turn on the oven and let it heat up to 350 degrees. As the oven is getting nice and warm, you can add the salt, sugar, and vinegar to a bowl along with the vegetables that you shredded up earlier. Toss it all together and combine it before setting it to the side.
2. Next, we can slice up the baguette into four pieces to use for this. Add these into the oven and let them get toasted in the oven. You only need to leave them there for around five minutes.
3. Take each of these from the oven and then cover with some of the hummus, the prepared tempeh slices, and the vegetables. Add some of your chosen herbs on top as well and then serve.

Nutritional values per serving

Calories 338
Carbs 40g - Protein 16g - Fats 11g

Curried Tofu Wraps

Prep time 35 minutes - Serves 4

What's inside:
- Quartered limes (2)
- Chapatis (8)
- Sliced garlic cloves (2)
- Sliced onions (2)
- Oli (2 Tbsp.)
- Tandoori curry paste (2 Tbsp.)
- Shredded red cabbage (.5)
- Dairy-free yogurt (4 Tbsp.)
- Mint sauce (3 Tbsp.)
- Tofu cubed (600g)

How to make this:
1. To start with this recipe, we want to mix together the yogurt, mint sauce, and cabbage. When this is well combined, we can set it to the side.
2. Toss together the tandoori paste with the tofu. Then add a bit of the oil to a frying pan. Add the tandoori tofu to the pan and let it cook for a bit to get all of the sides nice and golden. Take off the heat when this is done.
3. Then we need to use the same pan and add in the onions and garlic. Let these cook too.
4. After another eight minutes, add the tofu back to this pan and cook to heat back up.
5. You can follow the instructions on the package for warming up the chapatis and then fill these up with some of the tofu and the sauce that we made earlier.
6. Serve with a bit of lime and enjoy.

Nutritional values per serving:
Calories 497
Carbs 38g - Fat 25g - Protein 27g

Chapter 10: Snacks and Desserts

Chocolate Chip Muffins

prep time 15 minutes
serves 8

what's inside:

- vanilla protein powder (2 scoops)
- applesauce (1 c.)
- almond or nut butter (.5 c)
- almond flour (.5 c.)
- baking powder (1 tsp.)
- Chocolate chips (.5 c.)

How to make this:

1. Take the time to turn on the oven and heat it up to 350 degrees. Then take the time to prepare some muffin tins.
2. As the oven heats up you can take all of the ingredients from above and add into a big mixing bowl, making sure to stir around and get it well combined.
3. Divide this batter between your muffin tins as well as possible and then put it into the oven. A
4. After 15 minutes, the muffins should be done. Take them out and give them a few minutes to cool down before serving.

Nutritional values per serving

Calories 187
Carbs 15g
Fat 11g
Protein 7g

Black Bean and Chocolate Pudding

Prep time 2 hours
Serves 2

What's inside:

- Melted coconut oil (1 Tbsp.)
- Vanilla (1 tsp.)
- Salt (1 pinch)
- Medjool dates (2 pitted)
- Maple syrup (2 Tbsp.)
- Cocoa powder (.25 c.)
- Coconut or almond milk (4 Tbsp.)
- Black beans, cooked (1 c.)

Optional servings:

- Peanut butter
- Sliced banana
- Sliced strawberries
- Coconut whipped cream

How to make this:

1. To start, we want to drain and then rinse the black beans off so they are ready. Then take out the blender and add the beans inside.
2. Add in the rest of the ingredients here and then blitz to make them nice and smooth.
3. You can then pass this new mixture through a fine-mesh strainer so all of the extra pieces are taken out.
4. Scoop this mixture into some serving containers and then add to the fridge so that it can set and get thicker. This will take around two hours or more.
5. Serve chilled with some fruit on top if you would like.

Hazelnut and Chocolate Bars

Prep time 15 minutes
Serves 4

What's inside:

- Brown rice syrup (3 Tbsp.)
- Cashew butter (.25 c.)
- Almond milk (.33 c.)
- Unsweetened cocoa powder (.25 c.)
- Chopped hazelnuts (.25 c.)
- Vegan protein powder, chocolate (1 c.)

How to make this:

1. To start this recipe, take out a bowl and add in the hazelnuts, cocoa, and protein powder. Mix using your whisk to help combine well.
2. You can then continue on with this by adding in the brown rice syrup, cashew butter, and almond milk. Whisk to make them combined, but realize that it is going to start to turn into a dough and bit a bit sticky.
3. Layout some parchment paper on a tray and then add the dough to the middle. Press it out with a rolling pin or your hands.
4. Put this whole tray into the fridge to set for about four hours. Or if you need this to go faster, add to the freezer and leave it there for an hour and a half.
5. Slice this up into 8 bars and then serve.

Nutritional values per serving

Calories 296
Carbs 21.3g
Fat 14.2g
Protein 21g

Sweet Lentil Bites

Prep time 30 minutes
Servs 8

What's inside:

- Chopped almonds (.25 c.)
- Maple syrup (.5 c.)
- Almond butter (.5 c.)
- Shredded coconut (.25 c.)
- Pumpkin seeds (.25 c.)
- Cooking oats (1.5 c.)
- Salt
- Allspice (.5 tsp.)
- Cinnamon (.5 tsp.)
- Coconut oil (.5 Tbsp.)
- Green lentils (.75 c.)

How to make this:

1. Go through and prepare the lentils using one of your favorite methods to get it done. Then turn on the oven and let it heat up to 375 degrees. While that warms up you can use some parchment paper to line a baking pan.
2. Take the lentils that you just cooked and add to a bowl with the salt, allspice, cinnamon, and coconut oil. Mix it together well.
3. Pour this to that baking pan you prepared and spread them out before adding to the oven. About halfway through the cooking process, you can stir them around.
4. After 20 minutes, take the lentils out of the oven and give time to cool down.
5. Mix together the crushed almonds, maple syrup, almond butter, shredded coconut, seeds, and oats. Add the lentils into here and mix to combine.

6. Roll these all into some balls with the help of an ice cream scoop and then put them onto a plate. Set them into the fridge to harden for an hour and then serve.

Nutritional values per serving

Calories 264
Carbs 31g
Fat 12g
Protein 7.4g

No-Bake Treats

Prep time 20 minutes - Serves 8

What's inside:
- Brown rice syrup (.25 c.)
- Almond milk (2 Tbsp.)
- Vegan protein powder (.75 c.)
- Almond butter (.75 c.)
- Puffy rice cereal (4 c.)
- Vanilla (1 Tbsp.)
- Crushed almonds (.33 c.)
- Shredded coconut (.33 c.)
- Crushed hazelnuts (.33 c.)
- Salt (.25 tsp.)

How to make this:
1. Take out a nice baking dish that is square and add a bit of paper for baking inside. Set to the side for now.
2. Now we need to work with a pan, and we can heat it up on the stove. When it is set, you can add in the salt, almond butter, protein powder, almond milk, and brown rice syrup.
3. Let these simmer on a low setting until the ingredients start to bubble. Then add in the rice cereal and the vanilla, mixing these together until they are coated well.
4. Move this whole thing into that baking dish that you already prepared and then press down until it is an even thickness all around.
5. Sprinkle the top of this with some coconut and almonds and add to the freezer to let it firm. After an hour, you can take these out and slice into 8 pieces before serving.

Nutritional values per serving:
Calories 191
Carbs 13g - Fat 11g - Protein 9g

Zucchini Muffins

Prep time 40 minutes
Serves 8

What's inside:

- Quinoa, dry (.5 c.)
- Coconut oil (2 Tbsp.)
- Almond flour (1.5 c.)
- Chopped walnuts (.5 c.)
- Bananas (2)
- Applesauce (.5 c.)
- Maple syrup (.25 c.)
- Shredded zucchini (.5 c.)
- Vegan protein powder (1 c.)
- Dark chocolate chips, vegan (.5 c.)
- Almond milk (5 Tbsp.)
- Baking powder (2 tsp.)
- Cinnamon (.5 tsp.)
- Vanilla (.5 tsp.)
- Nutmeg (.5 tsp.)
- Water (.5 c)

How to make this:

1. Go through and prepare the quinoa using the instructions that are on the package. You can also turn on the oven to 400 degrees and then line a muffin pan and get that set up well too.
2. Take out a big bowl and mix together your baking powder, quinoa, walnuts cinnamon, salts, and nutmeg.
3. Take out another bowl that you can use and add the banans and mash it with a fork with the applesauce as well. then stir in the almond milk, protein powder, maple syrup, and protein powder.

4. Combine these two mixtures that we have been working with until they are nice and smooth and there are no lumps in it.
5. Carefully add in the chocolate chips now, as well as the zucchini that you shredded up. Add into the muffin cups, filling them about half the way up.
6. Add to the oven and let it bake for a bit. After 20 minutes, these muffins should be done. You can take them out of the oven and then let them cool down before serving.

Nutritional values per serving

Calories 354
Carbs 30g
Fat 19g
Protein 14g

Lemon Bars

Prep time 10 minutes - Serves 6

What's inside:
- Chia seeds (.25 c.)
- Pecan pieces (.25 c.)
- Raw cashews (.33 c.)
- Sunflower seeds (.33 c.)
- Pitted dates (2 c.)
- Vanilla protein powder, vegan (.5 c.)
- Organic lemon juice (2 Tbsp.)
- Salt (.25 tsp.)

How to make this:
1. Take out the chia seeds and soak them in some water for at least half an hour. When this is done, we can take the time to drain out any water that is left.
2. Then it is time to add the cashews, pecans, chia seeds, and the sunflower seeds into your own food processor. Make sure to pulse and mix these ingredients together until they make a mixture that is crumbly.
3. Add in the juice along with the salt and the dates. Continue to pulse all of these together while you add in your protein powder. We want the mixture to get chunky but still feel like dough.
4. When that happens, we can line a baking sheet with a bit of paper and then move the dough over to it. Use a rolling pin or your own fingers to press this out to make a thick square.
5. Add this whole pan to the freezer and let it stay there for at least 60 minutes, or until the chunk is nice and solid.
6. Take out of the freezer and slice into 8 bars before serving.

Nutritional values per serving:
Calories 272
Carbs 35g - Fat 11g - Protein 9g

Sunflower Protein Bars

Prep time 15 minutes - Serves 6

What's inside:
- Salt (.25 tsp.)
- Nutmeg (.25 tsp.)
- Cinnamon (1 tsp.)
- Old fashioned oats (1 c.)
- Puffy rice cereal (1 c.)
- Chocolate vegan protein powder (1 c.)
- Vanilla (2 tsp.)
- Maple syrup (.5 c.)
- Sunflower butter (.5 c.)

How to make this:
1. To start this recipe, bring out a bowl and add together the salt, nutmeg, cinnamon, protein powder, rice cereal, and oats. Set this to the side.
2. Take out another bowl that you can use and add in the maple syrup and the sunflower butter. Heat it up in the microwave for half a minute.
3. Take the mixture out of the microwave and mix the heated ingredients with the dry ingredients.
4. Stir this well and then add in the vanilla. Use a whisk to make sure that the lumps are gone and you have a nice and smooth mixture.
5. Spread this into a dish that is shallow and then line with some paper. Pack it down with a spoon to make sure that all of the air bubbles are gone.
6. Move to the freezer and let it sit for a bit. After about 20 minutes, we can take the dish out and slice into six bars before serving.

Nutritional values per serving:
Calories 188
Carbs 22g - Fat 6.8g - Protein 9.6g

Southwest Stuffed Bowls
Prep time 30 minutes - Serves 4

What's inside:
- Hummus (.25 c.)
- Dry black beans (1 c.)
- Dry chickpeas (.25 c.)
- Water or you can work with vegetable broth (1 c.)
- Chopped onion, purple (.5)
- Garlic powder (1 tsp.)
- Cumin (.5 tsp.)
- Paprika (.25 tsp.)
- Avocados halved (4)
- Salt (1 pinch)
- Lime juice (1 tsp.)
- Salsa (.25 c.)

How to make this:
1. Take the time to prepare both the chickpeas and the black beans using some of your favorite methods ahead of time.
2. Bring out a pot and heat it up on a higher temperature. Add either the vegetable broth or water. When these are warm, it is time to add in all of the spices, onions, chickpeas, and black beans.
3. When these are in, you can stir to combine all of the ingredients and then cook up the mixture so that most of the liquid is all gone.
4. After 15 minutes, this should be all done. In the meantime, you can sprinkle the halves of avocado with the salt and a bit of lime juice. You can serve these halves with some of the bean mixtures and then top with the salsa and hummus and enjoy.

Nutritional values per serving:
Calories 351
Carbs 33g - Fat 20g - Protein 10g

Brownie Bars

Prep time 15 minutes
Serves 3

What's inside:

- Chocolate vegan protein powder (2.5 c.)
- Cocoa powder (.5 c.)
- Quick style oats (.5 c.)
- Vanilla (1 tsp.)
- Nutmeg (.25 tsp.)
- Agave nectar (2 Tbsp.)
- Cold coffee that is brewed (1 c.)

How to make this:

1. Take out a baking dish that is square and line it with a bit of paper. Set this to the side for now.
2. Bring out a big bowl and then mix the dry ingredients together. When those are done, add in the cold coffee, nectar, and the vanilla, making sure that you stir this around so that the lumps are no longer there.
3. Then it is time to pour this batter into your dish, taking the time to press it down so it gets into the corners well.
4. Add this into the fridge so that it has time to get nice and firm. After four hours, it will be done. You can also add to the freezer to speed things up as this only takes about 60 minutes.
5. When that is done, take the dish out of the fridge and then slice into 6 pieces before serving.

Nutritional values per serving:
Calories 213
Carbs 17g
Fat 4g
Protein 27g

Chewy Butter Balls

Prep time 15 minutes
Serves 2

What's inside:

- Carob chips (1 Tbsp.)
- Puffy rice cereal (1 c.)
- Vanilla (1 Tbsp.)
- Almond butter (.25 c.)
- Vegan protein powder, vanilla (.5 c.)
- Maple syrup (2 Tbsp.)

How to make this:

1. Bring out a bowl and add inside the vanilla, almond butter, protein powder, and maple syrup. Mix until well combined.
2. Take the bowl and add it to the microwave. Cook and heat up until they are nice and melted.
3. Add in the puffy rice cereal along with the carob chips. Make sure to stir it all together so that it is nice and even one more time.
4. You can then line a sheet pan with a bit of parchment paper and then use a spoon to scoop out the mixture and make it into some small balls in your hands.
5. Press each of these firmly together to help prevent the crumbling and then add back onto the pan. Put into the freezer to set for about an hour. Enjoy when ready.

Nutritional values per serving

Calories 329
Carbs 25g
Fat 16.5g
Protein 21g

Carrot Cake

Prep time 10 minutes
Serves 4

What's inside:

For the cake:

- Vanilla protein powder (3 Tbsp.)
- Pecans (.5 c.)
- Raisins (.5 c.)
- Stevia (1 tsp.)
- Ground nutmeg (.25 tsp.)
- Cinnamon (1 tsp.)
- Orange zest (2 Tbsp.)
- Orange juice (2 Tbsp.)
- Ground almonds (.5 c.)
- Dried coconut (.5 c.)
- Carrots (2)

For the frosting:

- Water as needed
- Maple syrup (2 Tbsp.)
- Coconut oil (2 Tbsp.)
- Lemon juice (2 Tbsp.)
- Soaked cashews (2 c.)

How to make this:

1. To start with this recipe, we want to bring out our blender and add in all of the ingredients listed above for the cake inside. Pulse until this is nice and blended and then press the mixture into the pan you are using.

2. Then it is time to make the frosting we want to use. After cleaning out the blender add in all of the ingredients that we listed above for the frosting.
3. Pulse these in the blender until they are well mixed. You can add in some more water if you need to make it a bit smoother.
4. Use this to frost the cake and enjoy it right away.

Nutritional values per serving

Calories 779
carbs 45g
Fats 51g
Protein 35g

Protein Oat and Banana Balls

Prep time 5 minutes
Serves 4

What's inside:

- Banana (1)
- Vegan protein powder, vanilla (1 serving)
- Rolled oats (85 grams)

How to make this:

1. Bring out the blender and add in the protein powder and oats. Blitz these together until the oats are chopped, but you do not want it to be all the way smooth.
2. Add the banana into this and then combine to make a coarse but pliable dough.
3. When this is done, you can roll these into 12 balls and then add to the fridge and enjoy it when ready.

Nutritional values per serving

Calories 141
Carbs 24g
Fats 7g
Protein 6g

Protein Brownies

Prep time 20 minutes
Serves 9

What's inside:

- Vegan protein powder, chocolate (2 scoops)
- Cocoa powder (.25 c.)
- Almond butter (.5 c.)
- Bananas (3)

How to make this:

1. Take the time here to turn on the oven and let it heat up to 360 degrees. Then you can take the time to bring out a small cake pan and grease it all up.
2. Bring out a bowl and add in the nut butter. Add to the microwave and let it heat up until nice and smooth.
3. Take out a food processor and blender and add in the nut butter, protein powder, cocoa powder, and banana. Blitz these together until they are nice and smooth.
4. Pour this whole thing into that pan we prepared and add to the oven. Bake until the brownies are nice and firm.
5. After 20 minutes, the brownies should be done. Allow them some time to cool down all the way and then slice up.

Nutritional values

Calories 134
Carbs 15g
Fats 7g
Protein 7g

Oatmeal Raisin Cookies

Prep time 30 minutes
Serves 5

What's inside:

- Vanilla (.5 tsp.)
- Raisins (1 Tbsp.)
- Almond milk (.25 c.)
- Honey (1 Tbsp.)
- Raw oats (.5 c.)
- Agave syrup (.25 c.)
- Protein powder, vanilla (.5 c.)
- Natural almond butter (3 Tbsp.)

How to make this:

1. Add all of your ingredients except for the nuts, chocolate chips, and raisins, into the food processor. Blitz around to make a nice dough that we are able to mold with our hands. Then we can add in the toppings.
2. Divide this into five balls and then add into a baking tray that is lined with some baking paper. Press these down to make some cookies.
3. Turn on the oven and turn it up to 350 degrees. When this is ready, add the cookies inside and let them cook until they are nice and browned on top.
4. After 10 minutes, the cookies should be done. Allow them some time to cool down before you serve.

Nutritional values

Calories 211
Carbs 28g
Fats 7g
Protein 12g

CONCLUSION

Thank you for making it through to the end of *The Vegan Athlete*, let's hope it was informative and able to provide you with all of the tools you need to achieve your goals whatever they may be.

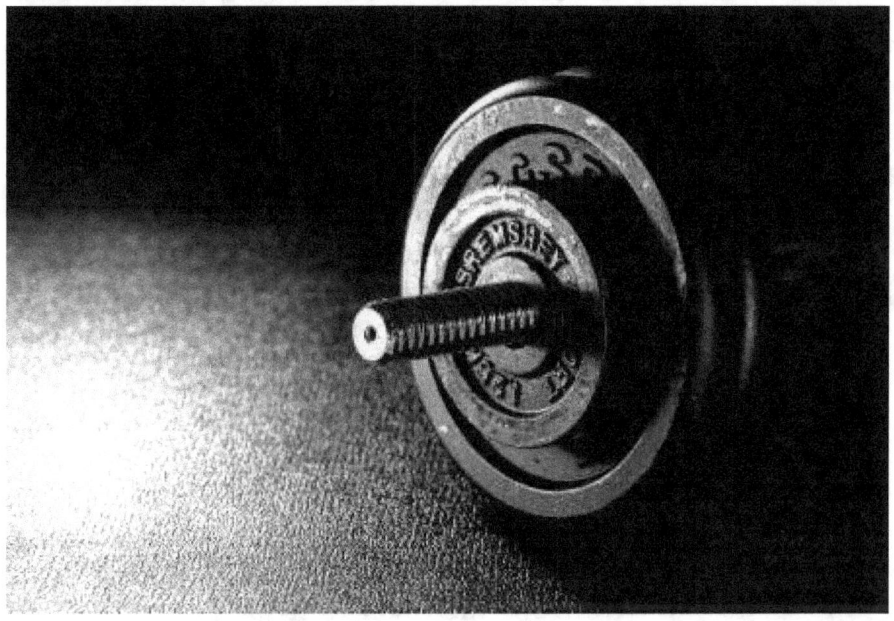

The next step is to start making your own meal plan and figure out what steps you need to follow in order to become a vegan on your own as an athlete. We took the time to talk all about the benefits of this great diet plan, and we even took a look at some of the basic foods that are going to help you get all of your nutrients when you are vegan. There are a lot of misconceptions out there about the vegan diet, but as more and more people learn about how healthy and wholesome it is, and even as more and more bodybuilders and athletes start to try it out and see results as well, it is likely that the rise in popularity will keep ongoing.

In this guidebook, we took the time to go through some of the basics that we need to know when we want to be a vegan athlete. We talked about the vegan before moving on to some of the basics of being an athlete and trying to make this diet plan work. We talked about the importance of protein and how we are able to get enough even on the vegan diet. We looked at some of the unique nutrient requirements of being on the vegan diet when we want to do an anaerobic activity, and how the vegan diet can help. And we even took a look at some of the basics that need to be met if a bodybuilder chooses to be on this kind of diet plan.

We also dived into some of the basics that are necessary for making meals that are vegan and athlete-friendly in the process. This is sometimes the hardest part of the whole thing because we worry about finding meals that are really delicious and good, but then also ones that are going to meet all of our nutrient requirements in the process. This guidebook has a ton of delicious and easy recipes that you are able to use to ensure that both of these requirements are met and you can follow this diet in the manner that you want.

There are so many benefits to going vegan as an athlete and it is so worth your time to learn more get started. This guidebook is going to be the tool that you need to help you there. When you are ready to work with this diet plan to help you get the best performance out of your athletics, make sure to check out this guidebook to help make that dream a reality in no time.

Finally, if you found this book useful in any way, a review on Amazon is always appreciated!

www.ingramcontent.com/pod-product-compliance
Lightning Source LLC
Chambersburg PA
CBHW070910080526
44589CB00013B/1249